. ACNE .

ANSWER

A STEP-by-STEP GUIDE
to CLEAR, HEALTHY SKIN

from SCIENTIFIC ORIGINS
to NATURAL, EASY,
EFFECTIVE SOLUTIONS

BY MARIE VÉRONIQUE NADEAU

This book is not intended as a substitute for the medical advice of physicians. The reader should regularly consult a physician in matters relating to his/her health and particularly with respect to any symptoms that may require diagnosis or medical attention. Although the author and publisher have made every effort to ensure that the information in this book was correct at press time, the author and publisher do not assume and hereby disclaim any liability to any party for any loss, damage or disruption caused by errors or omissions, whether such errors or omissions result from negligence, accident or any other cause.

Published by Bitingduck Press
ISBN 978-1-938463-57-0
©2016 M. Nadeau

For information contact:
Bitingduck Press, LLC
Altadena, CA
notifications@bitingduckpress.com
bitingduckpress.com

To Wayne, Wuzzle and Jenny
(and Fat Eddy, if she doesn't bite)

TABLE of CONTENTS

INTRODUCTION

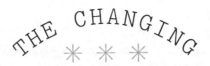

THE CHANGING
✳ ✳ ✳
FACE OF SKIN CARE

Dramatic changes are happening everywhere, from geopolitical alliances to economic upheavals to climate change. Now, cutting-edge news on the physics front tells us to stop being so universe-centric. We're no longer mere selves uniquely alone in a measly little universe. Instead, we inhabit a multiverse where literally anything is possible.

At the same time, microbiological research is uncovering multiverses far too small to see with the naked eye. Consequently, to get serious about skin care means to accept the immense complexity of these "miniscule" discoveries.

We generally regard skin as composed of three hardworking layers: dermis, epidermis and stratum corneum. Their jobs range from environmental protection/information gathering and maintaining proper temperature to immune system functions that protect us from disease. However, new research indicates that the vital role in defining our makeup, played by microbiota, also extends to our body's largest organ.

Thus, the fourth component of skin is its microbiome. This fourth layer is colonized by a diverse assortment of microorganisms, most of which are harmless or even beneficial. A few are pathogenic and can instigate acne formation.

Regarding the skin's surface as an ecosystem composed of various eco-niches gives us a different perspective on the treatment of acne. Microorganism colonization is driven by numerous factors. Endogenous host factors, like changes in hormone production that occur in different periods of our lives—particularly adolescence—are some of the main instigators of acne. Exogenous environmental factors, like overuse of antimicrobial soaps and anti-acne products, also contribute to acne formation, and in a way I believe can be cumulative.

The good news is that exploring these factors will highten our understanding of the underlying causes of acne—knowledge that will lead to unique and effective ways to treat it. That's what this book is about.

Acne Answer is divided into four sections, including a case history.

|| NOTE: IF TREATING YOUR SPECIFIC CONDITION IS ||
|| PRIORITY, JUMP AHEAD TO SECTION 2 ||

SECTION 1 Background and information

Chapters 1.1, 1.2 and 1.4 are in-depth explorations of the latest research findings about acne formation.

Chapter 1.3 is a playlet that breaks from the serious to convey a stunningly important message. You'll enter the microscopic world of Krobeville, and view your skin from your microbes' perspective. I hope you'll spend some time here and get acquainted with the microbes inhabiting the skin of our *Homo sapien* protagonists, Penelope and Keisha. It's your chance as host to get cozy with your own skin's microbial multitudes.

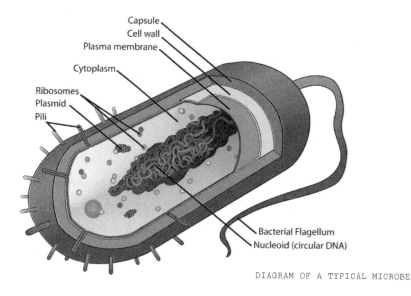

DIAGRAM OF A TYPICAL MICROBE

After all, each square centimeter of your skin averages about 100,000 bacteria. They're quite endearing and, truthfully, most of them just want to help. With just the tiniest bit of kindly encouragement, they'll work their little, um, plasmids, out for you.

Chapters 1.5 and 1.6 discuss alternatives to conventional methods used to control acne. We find that working with instead of against nature produces far better long-term results. Adults battling acne should not have to trade in their pimples for premature wrinkles. The win-win of alternative methods is specifically for them, helping skin stay younger-looking longer while acne is brought under control.

Chapter 1.7 covers our new understanding of what really causes rosacea. Chapter 1.8 is devoted exclusively to men's skin and its unique issues.

CASE STUDY Clara had clear skin with no problems until the age of 32. The onset of acne was very sudden and not accompanied by changes in diet. Follow Clara's step-by-step treatment path to success: clear, healthy skin.

SECTION 2 Treatment guidelines

Learn specific treatment routines tailored to who you are and your type of skin condition. Here you'll find guidelines for treating, topically and internally, men's and women's adult acne, acne vulgaris and inflammatory conditions including rosacea and hyperpigmentation. Consider this your all-in-one resource for treating acne and related conditions.

SECTION 3 New information supporting the future of skin care, including new approaches to treatments that represent a true break from the past.

Enjoy!

NEW

PERSPECTIVES

on ACNE

· SECTION ·
ONE

SEPARATING FACT FROM FICTION

DEALING WITH ACNE CAN BE EXTREMELY FRUSTRATING, and many of us struggle with it from teen years well into adulthood. Others won't encounter acne until later in life, many experiencing their first breakouts in their 30s or even later.

According to researchers at Massachusetts General Hospital, acne afflicts people across the age spectrum, for example the percentages of women with acne are 45% in ages 21-30, 26% in ages 31-40, and 12% in ages 41-50.

Acne vulgaris, ranging from the occasional breakout to crops of pimples that seem to last forever, is no longer considered exclusive to adolescents. Acne solutions, unfortunately, tend to be based on adolescent physiology, and with few choices adults too often settle for treatments that add insult to injury by simultaneously delivering poor results and accelerating the aging process.

All age groups deserve a shot at receiving effective treatments without dangerous side effects. Let's start by clearing up, so to speak, some of the misconceptions surrounding the causes of acne.

FICTION Your struggle with acne will lessen the older you get, and if you wait it out your skin will eventually clear up.

FACT Although acne vulgaris, or common acne, is accepted as an affliction that plagues most teenagers to some degree or another, adult acne actually affects 25% of all adult men and over 50% of adult women at some time in their adult lives. People can develop acne in their 20s, 30s, 40s and beyond, and it seems that dermatologists are seeing more adult acne patients than in previous decades. An article in the *International Journal of Cosmetic Science* in 2004 stated, "Recent epidemiological studies show that there appears to be an increase in post-adolescent acne, and that the disease is lasting longer and is requiring treatment well into the mid-forties."

FICTION Poor hygiene and poor diets are major causes of acne.

FACT Diet does play a big role, but whether vulgaris or adult, acne can be regarded primarily as a hormonal disorder. During puberty, a sharp rise in androgens like testosterone stimulates oil gland activity. Though both males and females can experience problems with acne as teenagers, severe or cystic acne is almost exclusively a male, androgen-related problem. Beyond puberty hormones start to favor the male over the female in the skin department. He starts to produce testosterone in amounts that keep his skin pimple-free *and* wrinkle-free. Ever wonder why men don't appear to age at the same rate as women? One reason is that testosterone creates thicker skin due to greater collagen density, slowing the appearance of wrinkles. Meanwhile, she starts the hormone rollercoaster. A sharp decrease in estrogen and rise in testosterone govern cycles of ovulation and menstruation, also seen in pregnancy, perimenopause and menopause. The result: adult women more than men can experience a worsening of existing acne or breakouts for the first time. Certain conditions like polycystic ovarian syndrome (PCOS) stimulate testosterone production, which leads to acne breakouts, while medications like steroids and birth control can interfere with normal hormone production.

FICTION The biggest contributor to acne is oily skin.

FACT Sebum production is the major contributor to most acne and may give skin a greasy look, but it does not imply truly "oily" skin. Blemish creation actually depends on a number of factors working in concert:

№ 1 FOLLICULAR EPITHELIAL HYPERFOLIATION

№ 2 PRESENCE, ACTIVITY AND STRAIN TYPE OF
PROPIONIBACTERIUM ACNES (P. ACNES)

№ 3 INFLAMMATION

№ 4 EXCESS SEBUM PRODUCTION

Sebum is a thick, waxy substance designed to lubricate the skin. Sebum production starts at puberty, and excess sebum production is related to testosterone production, which explains why so many teenage boys are afflicted with acne.

During adolescence, cell turnover rate can be higher then the normal 28-day cycle, resulting in excess skin cells that plug follicles. Sebum combines with excess skin cells, and before you know it, plugged hair follicles, called comedones begin to accumulate.

FICTION Get rid of *P. acnes* and you eliminate the problem.

FACT Everyone hosts *P. acnes*. In fact, healthy pores contain only *P. acnes*. Destroying *P. acnes* has been the mainstay treatment for more than 30 years with oral and topical antibiotics, particularly benzoyl peroxide, leading the pack. However, it's still not clear how *P. acnes* contributes to acne while being a major commensal of normal skin flora. Whether *P. acnes* protects the skin as a commensal[1] bacterium or functions as a pathogenic factor in acne, or both, remain burning questions of the 21st century.

Microbiologists[1] investigating the scene have suggested that there are different strains of *P. acnes*, some more virulent than others.

Some strains produce a biofilm that can increase stickiness and cause more pore congestion. A plugged pore with its high lipid content and low oxygen concentration makes an ideal home for *P. acnes*. The microbes multiply rapidly, and they release inflammatory substances that break down follicular walls to facilitate their spread. However, it's an individual's immune system response that appears to be the key to acne's progress from that point on.

FICTION One treatment fits all.

FACT Acne etiology is really incredibly complicated, and just as each person has a unique skin microbiome, an individual's immune system handles local microbial populations differently.

The part played by genetic factors, with some reactions to bacterial populations such as *P. acnes* hypersensitivity, points to immune system dysfunction. In another fairly common dysfunction the immune system is not able to efficiently kill and remove the bacteria, and the inflammatory reaction persists. This leads to the creation of cysts, pustules and, ultimately, scars.

FICTION Conventional treatments work well for all acne, regardless of age.

FACT It's easy enough to follow the logical progression from excess sebum production to plugged pores attracting bacteria to inflammatory responses resulting in pustules. Most conventional treatments attack *P. acnes*, assuming excess sebum production and skin cell hyperproliferation, the underlying contributory factors, are present. These hidden causes pertain to nearly all acne cases, but some essential processes at adolescence recede into the background for adults. In adulthood, cell turnover rate slows down, and inflammation rears its ugly head as a major culprit in skin aging. We must be aware of the varied underlying factors when treating individual cases.

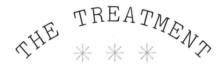

THE TREATMENT ✳ ✳ ✳
CONUNDRUM

All treatments base their solutions on one or more acne-contributing factors:

№ 1   FOLLICULAR EPITHELIAL HYPERFOLIATION

№ 2   PRESENCE, ACTIVITY AND STRAIN TYPE OF
      PROPIONIBACTERIUM ACNES (P. ACNES)

№ 3   INFLAMMATION

№ 4   EXCESS SEBUM PRODUCTION

Treating adult acne presents special challenges. Conventional treatments using benzoyl peroxide for example, control the acne-creating microbe *P. acnes*, but also dry the skin and generate free radicals, which aging skins cannot tolerate well. Indeed, most of the acne treatments currently available are designed for teenage skin, which has an almost infinite capacity to renew itself. Not so with adult skin. Let's explore how some popular treatments address various manifestations of acne—and their downsides.

COMEDOLYTICS/KERATOLYTICS

The first condition, follicular epithelial hyperfoliation, refers to cell turnover rate. During the teens, cell turnover rate can be higher than the normal 28-day cycle, resulting in excess skin cells that plug follicles. These microcomedones, without inflammation, look like whiteheads and blackheads. A common treatment involves reducing development of these microcomedones with topical comedolytics. Comedolytic products help the skin shed more effectively, preventing the pores from becoming plugged. Typical comedolytics are retinoids like Retin-A or beta hydroxy acids like salicylic acid.

TREATMENT DOWNSIDES

RETIN-A Overuse of Retin-A can cause skin irritation. Use of Retin-A during the day should be avoided as interaction with UV rays can exacerbate skin irritation.

SALICYLIC ACID The FDA has issued a warning against salicylic acid and benzoyl peroxide. Either one can, in very rare instances, cause severe allergic reactions[2] that can be life threatening. Symptoms include throat tightness, shortness of breath, wheezing, low blood pressure, fainting or collapse. If you have any of these symptoms, stop using the product and consult a physician. Isolated instances of hives and facial or body itching can also occur. If you experience hives discontinue use.

TOPICAL ANTIBIOTICS
and ANTIMICROBIALS

Over time, microcomedones can fill with *P. acnes* and become inflamed. The follicular walls swell, diffuse through tissue and produce enzymes that aggravate inflammation, thus attracting more bacteria. The upshot of all this activity can be a full-on breakout. The initial bacterial invasion sets up conditions for persistent cycles of infection and reinfection, which explains why many anti-acne treatments focus on fighting *P. acnes* with topical medications, or if that doesn't work, with oral antibiotics. Benzoyl peroxide remains effective against *P. acnes* and resistance does not develop. Topical antibiotics like erythromycin and clindamycin are often used in combination with BP.

TREATMENT DOWNSIDES

BENZOYL PEROXIDE (BP) It does bleach the skin, so it is recommended to take timeouts between courses of treatment to limit the photosensitization potential. **Always use a zinc oxide sunscreen, every day, rain or shine, while using products containing benzoyl peroxide.** BP can also cause severe allergic reactions in rare cases, and the FDA[2] advises discontinuing use if hives develop. Consult a doctor for any of the following symptoms: throat tightness, shortness of breath, wheezing, low blood pressure, fainting or collapse. BP is especially problematic when treating adult acne because it generates free radicals. Since most skin aging is attributed to free radical damage, it is clearly not a desirable treatment for older skin. Indeed, there is evidence from some *in vitro* studies that BP, in addition to generating free radicals, also promotes tumor growth. Topical antibiotics can cause irritation and contact dermatitis, and bacterial resistance is a frequent side effect, especially when used intermittently. In hopes of achieving better results, prescription acne medications often combine topical antibiotics with BP or retinoids.

ORAL ANTIBIOTICS

For more difficult acne cases, dermatologists continue to see oral antibiotics playing a role. This is a decision not to be embarked upon lightly by either party, and being aware of the risks is crucial.

TREATMENT DOWNSIDES

ORAL ANTIBIOTICS have a history of unfortunate side effects, including development of resistance by strains of *Staphylococcus aureus* and *Streptococcus pyogenes* that can have repercussions on health later on.

A recent report found "a three-fold increase in the prevalence of *Streptococcus pyogenes* in the oropharynx of those acne patients treated with systemic or topical antibiotics compared with acne patients not receiving antibiotics."[3]

ISOTRETINOIN, commonly known as ACCUTANE, has a long list of serious side effects including teratogenic and psychiatric effects. It is prescription-only and should be restricted to severe cases of acne that have not responded to other treatment protocols. Read on for alternative treatments that are both more effective and much safer—even with stubborn cases of acne.

REFERENCES:

1. *Journal of Investigative Dermatology* (2013) 133, 2152–2160; doi:10.1038/jid.2013.21; published online 28 February 2013: *Propionibacterium acnes* Strain Populations in the Human Skin Microbiome Associated with Acne

2. FDA: Topical Acne Products Can Cause Dangerous Side Effects, June 25, 2014

3. *American Academy of Dermatology*: "An update on the pathogenesis and management of acne vulgaris," by Julie C. Harper (July 2004) http://dx.doi.org/10.1016/j.jaad.2004.01.023

THE HUMAN SKIN MICROBIOME + ACNE

RESEARCH INTO MICROBIOMES OF THE HUMAN BODY, WHICH INCLUDE SKIN AND GUT, EXPANDS OUR ANTHROPOCENTRIC WORLDVIEW MICROSCOPICALLY AS WELL AS COSMICALLY.

It turns out that we are more our microbes than we are our human cells. In fact, microscopic life forms outnumber our own cells by nearly ten to one.

Much research has focused on the gut microbiome, including how negative consequences a course of antibiotics can affect gut health. Killing off beneficial bacteria can tip the balance in favor of over-colonization by pathogens, leading to intestinal dysfunction and chronic disease states[1]. A study[2] published in *Scientific American* suggests that our diet also has enormous impact on the gut microbiome. Populations of bacteria in the gut are highly sensitive to the food we eat—so sensitive, in fact, that changes in species variation and gene expression appear within three or four days following a major shift in diet.

The skin is another ecosystem, with three main eco-niches—sebaceous, moist and dry—that provide rich and diverse habitats for bacteria. While the skin microbiome is less studied to date, we can assume the same principle holds: maintaining microbiota balance is key to maintaining skin health.

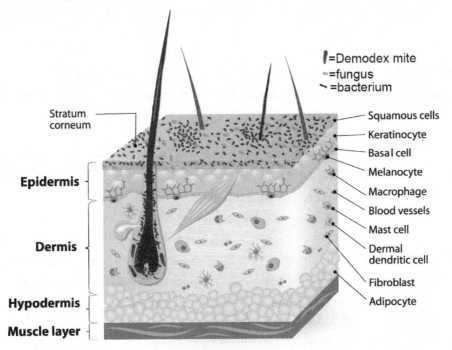

Skin microflora can be commensal (neutral), mutualistic or pathogenic, or in some cases, all three. An example of a mutualistic bacterium that can turn pathogenic is *Pseudomonas aeruginosa* (*P. aeruginosa*), which can cause dermatitis. However, *P. aeruginosa* also produces pseudomonic acid, which works against staphylococcal and streptococcal infections and inhibits growth of fungi like *Candida albicans*. So important is its role in maintaining balance that "removing *P. aeruginosa*[3] from the skin, through use of oral or topical antibiotics, may inversely allow for aberrant yeast colonization and infection."

Take the adage, "You are what you eat." Well, so are the bacteria living in your gut. With skin, the picture is slightly more complicated. Your skin reflects your gut health and what you eat to be sure, but the microbiota that have taken up residence on or beneath the skin's surface are also highly affected by what they eat topically. Feed them a daily diet of cleansers, serums, creams, lotions and the like, and you'll expose them to antimicrobials, either directly (antimicrobial cleansers or anti-acne products) or indirectly as part of the preservative moiety of a moisturizing cream, lotion or mist. It's the skin equivalent of taking a long course of antibiotics.

The implications for skin owners are huge. Skin is one of the human body's major ecosystems, home to a vast number of assorted microorganisms—1.8 square meters of diverse habitats populated by bacteria, viruses, fungi and mites.

Hosting all this teeming life is a huge responsibility when you think of it, but we humans take it for granted—until something goes wrong. As long as our mostly symbiotic microorganisms protect us against invasion by more pathogenic organisms, we go about our business.

However at the first sign of trouble (acne vulgaris, adult acne or rosacea), we're ready to nuke the dermal landscape with antimicrobial big guns like triclosan or benzoyl peroxide or antibiotics like clindamycin, doxycycline, erythromycin or tetracycline.

USE ANTIBIOTICS as a LAST RESORT

Follow a more moderate course to prevent antibiotics from disrupting the gut microbiome, and add probiotics and prebiotics to your diet to keep the microbiota balanced.

It's time to exercise the same caution with our skin microbiome. To kill every microorganism in the landscape—good, bad or indifferent—disrupts the balance of the skin's microbiome, ultimately causing more damage in the long term. Remember the Lorax? He spoke up for the trees. Now, I am here to defend the microbes. We can't live without them, and if we become better stewards on their behalf, they'll work hard to keep our bodies healthy and our skins glowing.

We may not know as much about skin flora and fauna as we do about those of the gut, but sufficient evidence suggests that alternatives to treating common skin conditions, like acne, can work very well—without conducting mass slaughter or doing long-term damage to your skin's ecosystem.

For proof that we're all in this together, meet the Who's Who in "Whoville" in the next chapter: *Zit Alors!*, a play in two acts and two epilogues.

~~~~~~

REFERENCES:

1. Genome Research 2010 Oct; 20(10): 1411–1419. doi: 10.1101/gr.107987.110 PMCID: PMC2945190 "Reshaping the gut microbiome with bacterial transplantation and antibiotic intake"

2. *Scientific American*:"The Gut's Microbiome Changes Rapidly with Diet," by Rachel Feltman, December 14, 2013

3. Skin Microbiota: a source of disease or defence? by A.L. Cogen, V. Nizet and R.L.Gallo, published in British Journal Of Dermatology, March 2008.(http://www.ncbi.nlm.nih.gov/pmc/articles/PMC2746716/)

ZIT ALORS!

A PLAY IN TWO ACTS AND TWO EPILOGUES

"A PERSON'S A PERSON, NO MATTER HOW SMALL."

— Zeke (*aka* Horton the Elephant) Dr. Seuss, *Horton Hears a Who!*

GLOSSARY

AEROBIC An aerobic organism or aerobe is an organism that survives and thrives in an oxygenated environment.

AEROTOLERANT Ability to survive in the presence of O_2 – as in facultative anaerobes that don't require O_2 for survival, but are not harmed by its presence.

ANAEROBIC An anaerobic organism does not require oxygen to grow.

COMMENSALISM A class of relationships between two organisms where one organism benefits from the other without affecting it.

FACULTATIVE ANAEROBE Organism that produces ATP (adenosine triphosphate) by aerobic respiration if oxygen is present, but can switch to fermentation when oxygen is absent (e.g., *Staphylococcus spp.* are facultative anaerobes).

GRAM-NEGATIVE A class of bacteria that do not retain the crystal violet stain—a counter stain re-colorizes the bacteria red or pink.

GRAM-POSITIVE Gram-staining distinguishes between different types of bacteria—gram-positive bacteria like *Staphylococcus* and *Streptococcus* take up the crystal violet stain.

MUTUALISM Both organisms benefit from each other.

PARASITISM One benefits while the other is harmed.

THE PLAYERS
A CAST WELL OVER 1 TRILLION

COMMON KROBZ IN THE HOOD:

PROPIONIBACTERIUM ACNES (P. ACNES): Rod-shaped, gram-positive, mostly commensal; part of flora of most healthy adult skin; aerotolerant

HABITATS: Skin surface, follicles

FOOD: Triglycerides in sebum

REPUTATION: Serious self-esteem issues; their contribution to causing

acne gives every microbe a bad name

SLOGAN: "Crobe, I'm busting out of this taco stand."

ATTIRE: Purple T-shirts and sneakers

CORYNEBACTERIUM: Rod-shaped, gram-positive; aerobic or facultatively anaerobic; group in the form of a 'V' as well as words or ideograms, occasionally pathogenic

HABITATS: Dry areas of skin

FOOD: Need biotin to grow

REPUTATION: Intellectuals to some, weirdos to others; hard to figure out

ENTERTAINMENT: Forming different words that appear to be Chinese

ATTIRE: Purple T-shirts, spectacles and pocket protectors

STAPHYLOCOCCUS EPIDERMIDIS (S.EPIDERMIDIS): Gram-positive cocci in grape-like clusters; part of normal skin flora; usually harmless, but will form biofilms on plastic devices like catheters "to keep the environment pure and plastic-free." If you buy their eco-friendly argument, they epitomize mutualism.

REPUTATION: Friendly, extroverted world travelers, found everywhere

ACTIVITIES: Hang out in clusters at film/music festivals and peace demonstrations; meditate on a mutualistic world

SLOGAN: "May you multiply in peace and love."

MUSIC: R&R, folk songs, disco

ATTIRE: Purple tie-dye T-shirts, capes, beads, sandals, rose-colored glasses

STREPTOCOCCUS MITIS (S. MITIS): Gram-positive coccus; forms chains; facultative anaerobe; part of normal skin flora; nutritionally fastidious; requires a rich medium to grow.

REPUTATION: Quick to take offense and somewhat paranoid; long known for giving the world mozzarella cheese and yogurt, not just sore throats

SONG: 'Chain Gang' by *S. thermophilus* (aka Sam "High Heat" the Cook)

DANCES: Conga lines and the cancan

SLOGAN: *"Zit alors!"*

ATTIRE: Designer clothes in shades of violet and lavender, and bow ties

ACINETOBACTER JOHNSONII: Gram-negative cocci in diploid chain formation; aerobic; commensal; part of normal skin flora

REPUTATION: Formerly thought to be meek and mild, turns out they have a mean streak.

SLOGAN: "Who, us?"

HABITATS: Moist and damp

ATTIRE: Hot pink T-shirts

MUSIC: Cajun and zydeco

OTHER KROBZ IN THE HOOD

STAPHYLOCOCCUS AUREUS (S. AUREUS): Gram-positive cocci clusters, commonly found on skin; not necessarily pathogenic, but can cause illnesses from mild to life threatening. Skin infections include pimples, impetigo, boils, cellulitis, follicultis, scalded-skin syndrome and abscesses. MRSA (methicillin-resistant *Staph aureus*) is caused by strains resistant to antibiotics used to treat staph infections.

Found mostly in hospitals, though a form called community-associated MRSA is spread by skin-to-skin contact. It often begins as a small pimple that grows into a painful boil and may proceed to become an abscess requiring surgical draining. Sometimes the bacteria remain confined to the skin, but can also burrow deep within the body, causing life-threatening infections in bones, joints, lungs and the heart. Necrotizing fasciitis (the flesh-eating syndrome) can also be caused by *S. aureus*, but other bacteria are frequently involved.

REPUTATION: The baddest, meanest and slipperiest of all Krobz in the Hood; their most-feared gang is the Krobz Brothers. Two resistance groups, MR (methicillin resistant) and VR (vancomycin resistant), form the Krobz Brothers' elite corps of terrorists; use sophisticated duck-and-cover techniques to defy containment, much to the dismay of their mutualistic and commensal neighbors. Ignoring pleas to "just get along" from the mutualism crowd, they're intent on killing everything in their path, epitomizing the phrase "opportunistic pathogen."

ACTIVITY: Taking over the world

SLOGANS: "Power to the pimple!" and "We want our fair share—and that's all of it"

SONG: MRSA, MRSA

ATTIRE: Dark purple leather jackets, boots, mirrored sunglasses

STREPTOCOCCUS PYOGENES (S. PYOGENES): Gram-positive, grows in chains; mostly pathogenic; mild infections include strep throat and impetigo; lateral spread into the deeper layers of the skin can cause erysipelas and cellulitis; *S. pyogenes* can also cause necrotizing fasciitis.

REPUTATION: Another nasty character, though not nearly as bad as *S. aureus* since they're still susceptible to penicillin

ACTIVITY: Playing boules

SLOGAN: "Yo, 'crobes, super glue!"

ATTIRE: Purple satin bowling shirts

THE X-RATED EXTRAS

DEMODEX FOLLICULORUM (DEMODEX F.): Mites living in hair follicles. 0.3-0.4 mm long; come out of hair follicles at night; eat skin cells, hormones, sebum and bacteria (like *P. acnes*) that collect in follicles.

REPUTATION: According to *P. acnes*, they are vampires and sluts; *Demodex f. mites* shun the light, and only emerge from their coffins at night to mate. And of course, they eat *P. acnes*.

SLOGAN: "Yes, we're having sex on your face. Deal with it."

ATTIRE: None—they go *au naturel* so they can have sex quicker.

DEMODEX BREVIS (DEMODEX B.): Mites living in sebaceous glands connected to hair follicles; smaller and much less adventurous than their larger cousin, they snuggle deep into sebaceous glands and stay put. Both species primarily hang out near the nose, eyebrows and eyelashes.

ACTIVITY: Cocooning

ATTIRE: They never go anywhere, possibly because they have nothing to wear

---

THE MACROBES

HOMO SAPIENS: Penelope and Keisha, best friends since third grade; share everything—even similar cases of acne vulgaris. PENELOPE, a budding actor, regards her breakouts as a tragedy transcending *Hamlet.* To KEISHA, the science nerd, they're an intellectual challenge that modern science has the tools to resolve. At least, eventually.

ACT ONE

SCENE 1: MACROBE SUBURBS

A tree-lined street in a suburban macrobe neighborhood.

Walking home from school, Penelope examines a large, inflamed pimple on the side of her nose.

PENELOPE: I can't believe this. Callbacks for *"Three Sisters"* are tomorrow. I swear, as soon as they said I was up for the role of Irina, this monster zit appeared. Popping up like a toadstool. And now it's the size of one. Ughhh!!!

KEISHA: Pen, you're going to be so good nobody's going to notice. The huge bump on your head from walking into that telephone pole is another story...

PEN: (BAM!) Ouch.

Pen rubs her forehead, and reluctantly puts away her mirror.

PEN: You'll be in the public eye too next week when you get that science fair award. Nerd paparazzi will be swarming—suppose you won't care if a zit the size of grapefruit pops up on your chin just in time for your mug shot?

KEISHA: You've got to be kidding. Science fair winners? Zits would only be conspicuous by their absence. But yeah, I admit I'd prefer not to have that two-nose look.

Pen shoots her a wounded look.

KEISHA: Oh, I didn't mean it that way. Look Pen, let's go to the drug-store—I've been reading up about zits and I know we can do something.

SCENE 2: DRUGSTORE

Pen and Keisha in front of shelves of anti-acne lotions. Keisha lectures, unconsciously mimicking her professor father.

KEISHA: You can put four causes of acne in a mnemonic: S for sebum, P for *Propionibacterium acnes*—that's *P. acnes* for short—hyperproliferation of skin cells, and inflammation. SHIP if you move stuff around a bit.

Keisha picks up jars and bottles, reads labels, sets a few aside for consideration.

KEISHA: (HOLDS LARGE BOTTLE) This face wash contains triclosan, a strong antimicrobial that kills *P. acnes*.

Puts it in the "keep" pile, then picks up more jars and a bottle.

KEISHA: Okay, this mask clears out your pores with salicylic acid. These cleansing pads have alcohol and salicylic acid, and this exfoliating wash has salicylic acid and glycolic acid. Any of these will wipe out dead skin cells and dried sebum collected in your follicles. (TAKES A DEEP BREATH)

The *P. acnes* lives in the sebaceous gland next to the follicle and feeds on the sebum it produces. As teens, we have lots of sebum, so *P. acnes* has plenty to eat. The population will outgrow its living space, especially if the follicle is plugged with dead skin cells and closed at the top. Then the microbes start releasing enzymes causing the cell walls to rupture, so they can move on to new follicles. The result is inflammation, primarily induced by *P. acnes*. After you finish purging your pores, apply the benzoyl peroside gel to kill off all the *P. acnes*. Put that on last, tonight.

PEN: (LOOKS UP) Boris has doubled since you started talking. I think you excited him with all this talk of rupture and inflammation. I need to know—can I wipe him out by tomorrow? My audition is at four.

KEISHA: Pen, come on. You just have to wait it out, and don't pick at it! You'll cause breaks in the skin driving the infection deeper and opening the gates for all other microbes to get in.

Here, get this coverup so it won't look so... red. I'll help you get started and even rehearse your lines with you for the umpteenth time. So stop worrying— it'll be fine.

SCENE 3: THAT EVENING. PENELOPE'S BEDROOM

Penelope in pj's, surrounded by an impressive selection of jars and bottles; puts on a layer of gel while on the phone to Keisha.

PEN: Ouch, ouch, ouch. Okay, this is the last layer! Is it supposed to burn like this?

(PAUSE) I know you said once was enough, but tomorrow is the big day ...

(PAUSE) Never mind. I can stand it. All done. I'm off to Moscow—I mean bed—I wish it was Moscow. Thanks, Keish—you're the best.

(FORCED CHUCKLE) Oh... Sleep knits up the raveled sleeve of care, and all that. Good night, sweet princess. I'm just soooo nervous!!!

Pen tosses, turns and finally falls asleep.

ACT TWO

SCENE 1: SCHOOL AUDITORIUM

Penelope recites Irina's opening speech from Chekov's "Three Sisters" to rows of empty seats, save for the conspicuous casting director, drama teacher and play director in front. Pen gazes out a fake window.

PEN: (WISTFULLY) To go back to Moscow. To sell the house, to make an end of everything here, and go off to Moscow ...

Abruptly, scene morphs into an empty classroom. Penelope assumes the half circle of folding chairs is occupied by her teachers, but a closer look reveals strangers. Strange-looking too, with rod-shaped bodies draped in purple, so small their legs dangle over the chair edges far above the floor. They wear baseball caps, each with a different insignia: P. acnes, S. epidermidis and S. mitis. P. acnes wears a purple T-shirt and sneakers; S. epidermidis wears a purple cloak and sandals; and S. mitis wears a ruffled lavender shirt and a deep purple bow tie. They glare at Penelope until she feels compelled to speak.

PEN: (RAMBLING) So, um... I'm sorry I choked up back there. I guess I was thinking of Moscow, Idaho and said Pocatello instead of Moscow the first time...not that I want to go back to Pocatello...though some actor was born in a trunk there...

P.ACNES: (HOLDS UP A HAND) Stop talking. Penelope is it? We are here to discuss recent activities that have—ahem—come to our attention. (REGARDS HER STERNLY)

Penelope looks scared; she's a good student, rarely gets into trouble, but not perfect.

(CONT'D) Nothing less than the wholesale slaughter of our relatives, friends and colleagues.

A murmur of angry agreement rises from the other two.

PEN: This must be a mistake. I abhor killing. I don't even eat meat—well, chicken and fish sometimes but...

P.ACNES: Stop talking! The slaughter was terrible to behold. I've never seen anything like it.

Nevertheless, those of us spared convened and agreed to contact You directly. Give You a chance to explain Yourself.

PEN: (VERY CONFUSED) Oh. Well. Thank you, I think. But wait—I don't know what you're talking about. Are you sure you have the right person?

Scans the room in hopes the real guilty party lurks nearby.

P. acnes closely examines an official-looking document.

P.ACNES: (ABRUPTLY) Your name is Penelope Angstrom, correct?

Pen nods.

Penelope Angstrom, You are charged with 200 billion counts of murder in the first degree. How do You plead?

PEN: What? Two hundred billion? This is a joke, right?

She forces a chuckle as the peculiar trio regards her in stony silence.

P.ACNES: How do You plead?

A profound silence, with exception of a pounding heart.

PEN (TINY VOICE): Uhhhh. Not guilty?

S. mitis looks triumphantly.

S.MITIS: (SPEAKS WITH A THICK FRENCH ACCENT) Oh la la. I told you she would not confess.

PEN: (NEAR TEARS) Confess to what? You're absolutely crazy—this is insane! I've done nothing!

S.EPIDERMIDIS: (MILDLY) Wouldn't rile him, dear. He can be a tad mean when he gets excited. Just confess. There's a good girl.

PEN: Confess to what? What is this, a kangaroo court?

S.MITIS: (SUSPICIOUSLY) What exactly is this Kanga Rue? Your criminal headquarters? (MENACINGLY) I can give You a sore throat, You know. Right before Your audition...

PEN: Oh no! I'm horrified of sore throats. I don't deserve it. This is all a mistake!

S.EPIDERMIDIS: I warned You, dear. Take my advice and cooperate.

(TURNING TO THE OTHERS) We agreed to show Her the devastation She caused.

PEN: What? What did I do? I'm innocent I tell you!

P.ACNES: You must answer for Your crimes, Pen.

S.MITIS: (POINTS A QUIVERING FINGER) No more *Monsieur* Nice Guy. I will give You impetigo and a sore throat. *J'accuse!*

Penelope bursts into tears. S. epidermidis intervenes.

S.EPIDERMIDIS: *Du calme,* S. mitis. We agreed to give Her a chance to see the devastation she caused. Besides, we'll need Her cooperation to defeat you-know-who. Right, everyone?

P. acnes nods, after dramatic shrugs and mouth splutters S. mitis also nods; they grow out of their chairs, stretching and expanding until they reach Penelope's size. The classroom walls blur and disappear.

SCENE 2: THE MICROWORLD OF PENELOPE'S SKIN

On the surface of Penelope's skin; the microworld town of Krobeville.

The group surveys a vast, arid landscape of crags, gullies and dried-up stream beds; random reddish mountains with yellow-white tops appear ready to erupt. The scene is post-apocalyptic; dead and dying bodies lie piled beneath twisted, blackened tree trunks as far as the eye can see. Body bags are hauled away with frantic activity; and pink-shirted bodies plead for water.

ACINETOBACTER JOHNSONII: Water! Please! We're dying of thirst!

To Penelope's right, groups form and reform into various patterns.

In the distance amasses a swarm of purple leather jackets. Small bonfires illuminate their backs and light up their scowling, fierce faces. The crowd can be identified by their jacket insignia. The biggest group wears the Krobz Brothers name; a smaller group are tagged as Resistance Fighters: methicillin; and a tiny group of youngsters identify themselves as Resistance Fighters: vancomycin.

NEW PERSPECTIVES ON ACNE

Every so often, someone starts a song—very raucously:

"...have MRSA, have MRSA, baby, have MRSA, have MRSA on me..."

Circling the large mob, lines of couples in flashy purple outfits appear to show solidarity by singing loudly and dancing in a conga line. They don't fit in, however, obviously singing a different song and marching to a different beat.

S.EPIDERMIDIS: In front of us are *Acinetobacter johnsonii.* They are commensals. They like moisture so you can imagine their suffering. And the bonfires are spreading.

S.MITIS: All Your fault. *Peut-être* I will give You erysipelas along with the impetigo and the sore throat.

S.EPIDERMIDIS: To your right are *Corynebacterium,* also friends and commensals. They form words in a mysterious code we've not been able to break.

They are very strange—even stranger than our sometime-friend here.

S.MITIS: (DREAMILY) Cellulitis, necrotizing fasciitis...

S.EPIDERMIDIS: Don't mind him. He's bluffing. Actually all he can do is make cheese.

S.MITIS: (INDIGNANTLY) ALL?

(GROWS LOUDER) You call that ALL?

S.EPIDERMIDIS: (IGNORES HIM) The real threat comes from that group ahead of us.

PEN: The ones singing in a conga line?

S.EPIDERMIDIS: The ones in purple Resistance jackets, singing. Their crowd is growing bigger by the second.

(SHUDDERS) The conga line in purple shirts is *Streptococcus pyogenes,* who are the cruel cousins of *Streptococcus mitis* here. In truth, *S. mitis* is a softie as long as he gets enough to eat.

S. epidermidis gives S. mitis a hug.

S.MITIS: Speaking of food, I am very, very hungry. I must go and check our food supplies, which have been sadly depleted by—Her.

(TURNS TO PENELOPE) I beg of You—come to Your senses and one day I hope to have You as my guest at the Lacto-Bacilli Club. It's the only club in the world where millions dance the cancan together.

(PAUSE) I would kiss Your hand but I am still too angry. *A plus tard,* 'crobes.

Scurries quickly away, with a twitching motion.

S.EPIDERMIDIS: Odd fellow; not our type, but he volunteered for this mission.

PEN: Hey! Did he just call us retards?

S.EPIDERMIDIS: No, no. It's just how he talks. His cousins, *S. pyogenes*, are much, much worse. I mean, vicious. But we must watch out for *Staphylococcus aureus*. (WHISPERS THE WORD) Pathogens.

PEN: I've heard of *Staph aureus*. My friend did her science project on MRSA. (PROUDLY) She won first prize!

S.EPIDERMIDIS: That's good, dear. Good. *P. acnes* can take over from here, and without further ado I must leave. I have millions of funerals to attend. Indeed I am officiating at most of them. (SIGHS AND PATS PEN'S HEAD) I will ask our comrades to forgive You. I really don't think You knew what You were doing.

PEN: (NERVOUS LOOK TO P.ACNES) Can't you come with me?

S.EPIDERMIDIS: Oh, no dear. You wouldn't want that. We don't inhabit the same places as *P. acnes*—unless there's a disaster.

Glides away to join clusters of mourners who suddenly appeared.

P.ACNES: Later 'crobe—thank you for your help!

P.EPIDERMIDIS: Peace, love and multiply!

P.ACNES: (TURNS TO PEN) Let's get out of here. I can't stand the sight of this devastation another nanosecond.

He grabs Pen's hand, leading her to a large cavern with downward-sloping walls. A huge tree trunk flanks one side. P. acnes decends, gripping Pen's hand so she's forced to follow.

PEN: Where are we going?

P.ACNES: Home. Home at last.

SCENE 3: KROBEVILLE UNDERGROUND. INSIDE SEBACEOUS GLAND

P. acnes pulls Penelope into a warm, cozy room with pink walls. Many just like him sit at a long table, plates piled high with what looks like lumps of grease.

P.ACNES: These are my roommates. Roomies, this is Penelope.

They look up, leave the table to crowd around P. acnes, patting him on the back. They eye Pen shyly, but steer clear of getting too close.

ROOMIES: Welcome back, 'crobe. 'Crobe, great job. Our hero....

P.ACNES: I need to speak with the top brass. A group meeting in the auditorium in five, pass it on. This way, Penelope.

They follow a long corridor, pearing in rooms with many diners sitting at long tables. P. acnes shouts out greetings, but doesn't slow his pace till he reaches double doors at the end of the hall.

P. acnes and Pen step onto a vast auditorium. A raised stage at the end is occupied by important group strutting about in purple military uniforms.

PEN (GASPS): Wow, this is like the biggest theater I have ever seen. What's the maximum seating?

P.ACNES: Oh, it's small. Only ten million, give or take.

Goes up to the military person with the most medals, salutes, clicks his heels.

General. Here She is. (PAUSES FOR EFFECT) Mission accomplished.

P. acnes steps back. General acnes is very fat and quite red in the face. He nods at Penelope. Looks back over to P. acnes.

GENERAL ACNES: Well, done, lad. We never thought you'd make it back, but here you are. What do you have to report?

P.ACNES: Sir, it looks like troop movements massing on the surface. They may be preparing an attack. At least several billion already in formation.

GENERAL ACNES: Have you explained the situation to our Host?

P.ACNES: Not yet General. I wanted everyone here.

Meanwhile, the auditorium has filled to capacity. The spotlight is on P. acnes.

He steps to the front of the stage.

P.ACNES: My 'crobes!! Welcome everyone. It's good to be home.

His announcement is met with cheers and whistles that go on for a long time.

P.ACNES: And now I am honored to present our Host, Penelope.

The spotlight switches to Penelope who blinks, then gives a tiny wave to the crowd. The crowd goes silent.

PENELOPE: (MUTTERS TO HERSELF) Wow, an actor's worst nightmare. A crowd of millions staring at you in hostile silence.

P. acnes clears his throat; spotlight mercifully returns to him.

P.ACNES: Penelope, it's time to explain why we brought You here.

PENELOPE: Am I on trial?

P.ACNES: No. We think S. epidermidis was right. You didn't know what You were doing. We've brought You down here in front of everyone to explain what You've done, the consequences of what You've done, and what You can do save us all.

Please, sit.

P. acnes offers her a chair on stage, then begins to draw on a large whiteboard.

PENELOPE: This feels strangely familiar. You sort of remind me of Keisha. Or maybe her dad.

P. ACNES: It's like this.

(DRAWS A BEAUTIFUL LANDSCAPE OF TREES, PLANTS, AND BUSY STREETS FULL OF PEOPLE)

This was the surface of Krobeville—before You firebombed us. You saw for Yourself what it looks like now.

PENELOPE: What are you talking about?

P. ACNES: The chemical warfare You visited on us very recently. You saw it—on the surface. It was a massacre.

PEN: (THE LIGHT DAWNS) Oh, the acne treatments! Is that what you're talking about? I'm actually the same size as you? Where am I anyway? This is all very down-the-rabbit-hole-ish.

P. ACNES: You're underground. In Pilosebaceous Unit Number 4014, Gland Number 13 to be exact.

PENELOPE: And you all are, uh...

P. ACNES: (PROUDLY) Kingdom: Bacteria, Phylum: Actinobacteria, Order: Actinomycetales, Family: Propionibacteriaceae, Genus: Propionibacterium, Species: *P. acnes.* At your service.

Bows grandly, with a flourish.

PEN: So, you guys are, um, microbes? Whoa wait, I remember Keisha telling me about *P. acnes.* Aren't you the ones giving me zits? You're responsible for Boris, the zit as big as my foot!

She straightens and a glint of defiance appears in her eyes as she continues.

And I killed a few of you? But, what do you expect? You're pathogens.

CROWD (ROARING IN ANGER): Did you hear what she called us? Pathogens???!!!! A few, She says! *etc.*

P. ACNES: Please settle down, 'crobes. She doesn't understand. (TO PEN) We're not totally to blame. If you hadn't done all the wrong things this situation would never have happened. And now that you've killed so many of us, *Staph aureus* is threatening to take over. That triclosan crap you've been using? You know what it kills? Everything but *S. aureus,* that's what.

S. MITIS: (SHOUTS FROM AUDIENCE) And *voila!* You will get boils!

There are shouts of agreement mingled with, "who let that guy in?"

P. ACNES: 'Crobes! 'Crobes! Quiet down! S. mitis was on our mission with us, my 'crobes. And he's right. Too much triclosan causes so much damage to all of us commensals and mutuals that we're overwhelmed. Then the pathogens take over. The REAL pathogens, not us. You saw them up there, they're getting ready to make a move. And believe me, you're not going to like what they do to your skin.

PEN: But are you pathogens or not?

Audience erupts into boos and hisses.

P.ACNES: Stop it! That is no way for guests to behave. Remember who She is! Besides, it's a fair question. She's just repeating the cruel lies from consumer brainwashing.

He goes back to the whiteboard.

(DRAWS A FOLLICLE)

Under normal circumstances we help your skin stay healthy. We eat sebum, which we hydrolyse into free fatty acids that rise to the surface, keeping skin lubricated, and at a low enough pH for *S. aureus* and *S. pyogenes*, who prefer higher pH numbers to stay away.

(DRAWS A PLUGGED FOLLICLE)

But if you produce so much sebum and so many skin cells that we can't maintain, things go haywire. Especially if the follicle exit gets plugged at the surface.

Here we are in our follicle, working away to secrete the digestive enzymes that keep everything humming along, but if the system overloads we, well, we rupture the follicular walls and inflammation sets in. Something you'd rather not have happen. We don't like it either, believe me; we'd rather just keep a

nice status quo with everything balanced. Inflammation is only a problem when things get out of balance.

We call it global warming. It attracts the bad guys like *Staph aureus* and *Strep pyogenes,* and before you know there's pus and swelling, more inflammation and a big, ugly mess on your face.

(DRAWS A PUSTULE)

PEN: Ew. That is really, really gross. Hey, we have global warming too.

P.ACNES: That so? It's a small world— no matter how big it gets.

Anyway, I wanted to bring you here because when we saw the damage you were doing, we knew we had to act before matters got completely out of hand.

(DRAWS A BOIL ON A NOSE)

P.ACNES: Continue what you've been doing, here's what will happen.

PEN: Eee-ewww. Boris the Pimple is bad enough.

P.ACNES: You don't want to go from Boris Badenough to Boris the Boil. There goes your career, am I right? Heh, heh, my little joke...

PEN: Oh all right. So I am assuming you have an answer?

P.ACNES: Ah! So glad you asked. To avoid career death, follow these simple steps.

(WRITES ON BOARD) *Step One: STOP THE RANDOM KILLING*

(DRAWS A TRICLOSAN CLEANSER WITH A CROSS THROUGH IT)

Cheers and whistles from the audience.

P.ACNES: A high dose of triclosan kills everything: us, *Staph epidermidis, Acinetobacter, Corynebacterium, Staph aureus,* your own skin cells—you name it. And if you use it enough, a state of affairs develops called microbial dysbiosis. The good 'crobes don't recover in time or in sufficient numbers to keep the pathogenic 'crobes in check. The normal balance is disrupted.

The result: (DRAMATIC PAUSE) microbial dysbiosis.

Looks at Penelope.

P.ACNES: Do You follow me so far?

PENELOPE: Oh hey, no problem. I'll just call you Keisha from now on...

P.ACNES: Fine. I believe her own mission-impossible team is visiting her right now.

PEN: Oh man, I'll bet she's enjoying it. Not being sarcastic, 'crobe, I mean it. She's seriously loopy about micro-organisms. According to her dad, I'm the stage-struck one; Keisha is the 'crobe-struck one.

P.ACNES: I am going to infer from Your remarks that I should keep the next part short. But it's really import-ant that You understand that we are in this together.

(SHORT PAUSE) Ahem. Large num-bers of gram-positives like *Streptococcus* produce factors that inhibit the growth of similar strains—for example our friend, Strep mitis, can produce bac-teriocins against closely related strains like *Strep pyogenes.*

Strep mitis jumps up and yells.

S.MITIS: Bravo! Bravo to me—I am the mighty mitis!

He struts and thumps his chest until audience members pull him down.

P.ACNES: Uh yes, thank you, *S. mitis*—good work. The other member of our mission impossible team, who can't be here with us, *S. epidermidis*...

PEN: Why can't she be here?

P.ACNES: She works on the surface. If she starts going below, you know your follicle is in trouble. But on your skin's surface she is very instrumen-tal—keeping everything in balance by producing various types of bacterio-cins. Her team plays a huge role in fighting off pathogenic attack.

P.ACNES (TO AUDIENCE): Let's hear it for *Staphylococcus epidermidis!*

The auditorium rings with cheers.

P.ACNES: Let's reinforce our role in

fighting pathogens once more. Free fatty acids are produced by lipases that we secrete by hydrolyzing sebum triglycerides. The free fatty acids on the skin's surface contain natural antimicrobials to keep pathogens in check.

(DRAWS A GRAPH)

(CONTINUES) Which gets me to the second step.

PEN: Oh, whew!

P.ACNES: (WRITES ON BOARD) *Step Two: GIVE YOUR SKIN THE RIGHT OILS*

(DRAWS AN OIL-FREE MOISTURIZER WITH A LINE THROUGH IT)

P.ACNES: It's so important to give your skin the right oils. Free fatty acids have antibacterial activity against several gram-negative bad guys, lauric acid and palmitic acid enhance the skin's immune system, and oleic acid has proven to be effective in containing MRSA infections.

(TAKES DEEP BREATH) There's more: linoleic acid, an omega-6 essential fatty acid, keeps sebum from clogging follicles and prevents comedo formation. As long as your follicles are clear, you can prevent the conditions that cause acne.

It's that simple. Sunflower, borage, grape seed and rosehip seed oils are high in linoleic acid. (PAUSES TO THINK)

And don't forget linolenic acid—an omega-3 essential fatty acid. It reduces inflammation and again, breaks the chain of events that creates Boris and his like.

PEN: No kidding! And to think they kept telling us to use oil-free stuff.

P.ACNES: (SHAKES HIS HEAD) So wrong. So criminally wrong. Now, (WRITES ON BOARD) *Step Three: ASK YOUR MICROBES*

This relies on your intuitive side, so as an actor I think you may find the concept easy to grasp ...

P. Acnes is approached by a minion bearing a note.

P.ACNES: Oh, pardon me.

P. acnes reads the note and moves to the front of the stage.

(STAGE WHISPER) Go to your shelters everyone. We've completely lost track of time.

Everyone begins filing out of the auditorium in an orderly fashion, careful to be very quiet.

PEN: Um, what's going on?

P.ACNES: Shhhhh. *Demodex folliculorum* is waking up.

PEN: Who?

P. acnes grabs her and throws her into a recess in the wall of the auditorium, then covers her with his body, signaling her to remain quiet. He's just in time.

Penelope peeks over P. acnes' shoulder and sees a humongous monster, about the size of a football field, gliding past. A ring of tentacles grows out of one end, which Penelope assumes is its head. Or heads. It slurps up a few thousand microbes who didn't get out of the way fast enough as it glides along the main corridor towards the exit.

As it oozes out the exit, a huge, gloppy, popping noise signals the microbes to emerge out of hiding.

PEN: Yuck—and double yuck! What was that thing?

P.ACNES: Demodex folliculorum. It lives here, but only comes out when it's dark. It's a giant spider.

PEN: How awful. You have to live with it? No way you can get rid of it?

P.ACNES: Did you see the size of that thing? Anyway, it's just life, you know. Though I can't imagine what a paradox it would create if it ate You. I mean, You are our Host.

PEN: Yeah, hmmm. I guess maybe it would get really big, and I'd wake up tomorrow as a giant spider. There's a story like that, only G. Samsa became a cockroach.

P.ACNES: That genus and species eludes me. What happened to him?

PEN: He died. It was a sad story. No happy ending.

P.ACNES: Unlike this story, right?

PEN: Right. Well I promise to follow your advice.

P.ACNES: You can do more things too. But read the rest of the book first.

PEN: Won't I see you again?

P.ACNES: Hey, we'll still be here, keeping everything running smoothly. But You'd better go—not back to the surface—come this way. When the spiders are out there mating even the Krobz commando squads stay away.

P. acnes shakes her hand and the others cluster around.

(CONTINUES) Just twirl three times and...

Penelope is swept up in to a vortex.

PEN: (CALLS BACK) My 'crobes! Goodbye, dear little 'crobes. I promise to be the best Host ever! And P. acnes and S. mitis—thanks to you I've seen the mites... I mean 'light.' Please give S. epidermidis a big hug. Good-bye!

'CROBES (WAVING THEIR LITTLE HANDS, SHOUTING IN UNISON): Good-bye, Penelope! Good-bye, dear Host! Au revoir! Stay in touch! Be kind to us! We love you, we have no choice! Etc.

As she waves the 'crobes shrink till they're just specks with tiny, tinny voices and disappear altogether.

Next morning. Keisha and Penelope meet on the way to school; speak excitedly at the same time.

KEISHA/PEN (SIMULTANEOUS):
I had the most amazing dream...

They look at each other and laugh.

PEN: You go first.

As they walk, Keisha talks animatedly.

KEISHA: I figured it out, Pen! *Corynebacterium* send code messages in the form of molecular structures, and signal what they need. What tipped me off was this:

(DRAWS LINOLEIC ACID MOLECULE)

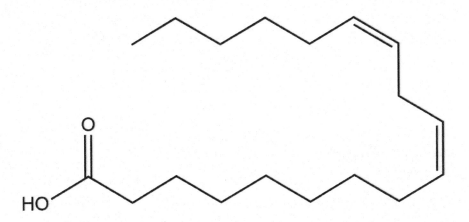

(PAUSES) That's how I knew what they needed. Other microbes sent distress signals by creating inflammation. It's all a beautiful dance of chemical interactions, Pen, coordinated to the trillionth of a second by a thousand different species—and that's just on one square centimeter of skin! Multiply that by a hundred trillion and...Indescribable! I felt like I was listening in on the music of the spheres. Oh, and you know how *Corynebacterium* make a pattern that looks like a V?

(PAUSES) Guess what that means— it's so breathtakingly simple.

PEN: Umm. V for victory? S. epidermidis would say, "V for peace and love."

KEISHA: Exactly! Those are other words for what *Corynebacterium* are trying to tell us. 'V' stands for homeostasis, of course. When everything is in balance they give us a V sign. I can't wait to tell Dad!

They walk along in silence, each overwhelmed by their own thoughts.

EPILOGUE

THREE MONTHS LATER

SCENE 1: SCHOOL DRAMA THEATER

Audience rises and cheers. Penelope bows, accepts a bouquet from adoring fans.

SCENE 2: BACKSTAGE

KEISHA: I am so proud of you, Pen. You were far and away the best one in the whole play.

KEISHA'S MOM: (HUGS PEN; LOOKS ON FONDLY) It's been a special year. Both you girls had dreams come true.

(TURNS TO PEN AS SHE REMOVES HER MAKEUP) Your skin is lovely, dear. All cleared up.

Turns to her daughter, then continues.

You know, now that you're not so anxious, neither one of you is breaking out any more. Have you noticed? It's the power of positive thinking.

Keisha's mom wears an elaborate velvet purple cloak, exuding serene confidence *that reminds Penelope of the little creature whose spirit is still with her, though she may be too small for Penelope to see.*

PENELOPE: Just wait till summer. Keisha cracked the code of *Corynebacterium* and she's off to the Young Scientists Camp in Cambridge...

Keisha's Dad beams.

PEN: And I get to act in the Summer Workshop—Miranda in *The Tempest*! My absolute favorite play.

(THEY FLASH EACH OTHER THE "V FOR HOMEOSTASIS" SIGN AND GRIN)

The inhabitants of Krobeville also celebrate their Hosts' triumphs across various facial landscapes.

SCENE 3: ABOVE & BELOW SKIN SURFACE

Random locations on and deep below the surface of the girls' faces.

At the Lacto-Bacilli Club millions of Streptococcus mitis dance the cancan. In moist areas, Acinetobacter johnsonii sing, fiddle and twirl to Cajun honky tonk.

S. epidermidis and her staff flash-mob dance to disco. S. aureus perform their when-we-behave-ourselves dance, boots thumping and rocking out. Surrounding their group are long chains of S. pyogenes kicking their legs lustily to strains of samba. Outside of town where it's dark, Demodex folliculorum hold a love-in, mating madly to a Haight-Ashbury soundtrack.

Deep underground in the auditorium of Pilosebaceous Unit Number 4014, Gland Number 13, P. acnes plays the wizard in The Tempest *before a packed house. Scanning an audience of multimillions, he repeats the lines that stand the test of any time and any size.*

PROSPERO ACNES: We are such stuff as dreams are made on, and our little lives are rounded with a sleep.

And in remote dry, deserted locations, Corynebacterium form Vs of homeostatic happiness while a choir sings Beethoven's "Ode to Joy." Music swells to fill their world, so vast to them, so tiny to us, but a neverending miracle to all, big and small, privileged to be a part of it.

EPILOGUE to the EPILOGUE

NARRATOR: Deep in Krobeville we find Zeke, an *A. pachydermis* (*Awesome pachyderm*), a soon-to-be-discovered animal, tiny by macrobe standards yet colossal by Krobeville measure, likely belonging to the rotifer class.

Zeke lazes upstream, scooping in microalgae with the tiny wheels on his head when he hears a wee voice coming from a fungus named Malassezia pachydermatis. With his cilia he carefully picks up the fungus, safely storing it in his trunk so no harm comes to it.

And on it goes ...

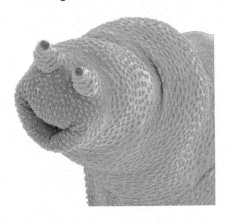

NARRATOR: (CONT'D) If anyone dares ask him what he thinks he's doing, Zeke staunchly replies: "A PERSON'S A PERSON, NO MATTER HOW SMALL."

– Dr. Seuss, *Horton Hears a Who!*

ZEKE, A POSSIBLE LIKENESS

WHAT CAUSES ACNE

P. acnes gave Penelope the story of acne from a microbe's point of view. Now let's look at the full picture of what actually happens on and below the surface of your skin.

ACNE FORMATION IS USUALLY ATTRIBUTED TO FOUR CAUSES:

№ 1 EXCESS SEBUM PRODUCTION

№ 2 FOLLICULAR EPITHELIAL HYPERFOLIATION

№ 3 OVER-COLONIZATION OF
     PROPIONIBACTERIUM ACNES (*P. ACNES*)

№ 4 INFLAMMATION

All this activity occurs deep in the hair follicle, long before anything shows on the surface.

PIMPLE PRODUCTION
STEP BY STEP

1. HORMONE IMBALANCE → EXCESS SEBUM PRODUCTION
Your sebaceous gland is situated alongside the hair follicle. Ideally the sebum it produces travels along the hair shaft to the skin's surface, where it forms part of the lipid barrier that both lubricates and protects skin against environmental assault. Because sebum production is hormone-dependent (testosterone being the main culprit), at certain stages in life like puberty, too much sebum is produced due to hormonal imbalances. Most of the sebum travels to the surface, however some remains lodged in the follicle.

2. TOO MANY SKIN CELLS → CONGESTION Cell turnover rate—
the time it takes a skin cell to be born in the basal layer, move to the top layer and become a keratinocyte (dead skin cell)—is about 28-30 days. Producing too many skin cells is common during puberty and with the skin disorder, psoriasis. Skin cells and assorted debris can collect in the follicle along with sebum, furthering congestion.

3. *P. ACNES* → MICROBIAL OVER-COLONIZATION *P. acnes* is
aerotolerant and can be found on the surface of your skin, but prefers living in a low-oxygen environment. For example, deep within a plugged follicle, *P. acnes* uses sebum as its primary food source, and as long as the pore isn't clogged *P. acnes* does not directly cause damage to the skin. In fact, healthy pores contain only *P. acnes*, which hydrolyses sebum into free fatty acids and propionic acid, aiding in proper skin barrier function. This happy state of affairs changes when the pore becomes clogged and a closed comedo forms. *P. acnes* makes more room for its ever-growing population by releasing enzymes that damage follicular walls. The damage clears the way for other microbes, including *Staphyloccocus aureus*, *Staphyloccocus epidermidis* and even some substrains of *P. acnes* that form sticky clumps known as biofilms.

All this gatecrashing results in infection followed by inflammation—when most of the serious problems start. In fact, the inflammatory process of the immune system is responsible for most of the damage caused by acne.

4 . DYSFUNCTIONAL IMMUNE RESPONSE → INFLAMMATION

The immune system reacts to the presence of *P. acnes* by sending in a flood of white blood cells. Skin that's extra sensitive to the microbes may overreact by producing large amounts of inflammatory cytokines, which induce white blood cells, releasing destructive enzymes and free radicals into the site of the infection. A vicious cycle ensues as more cytokines are released to repair mounting damage.

Another dysfunctional immune response occurs with individuals having a defect in their white blood cells' ability to kill the bacteria after eating them. The white blood cells continue to secrete inflammatory cytokines until they die. The bacteria can sometimes escape and continue proliferating. It's a mess. To really get the picture, take a close look at a healthy hair follicle alongside infected ones.

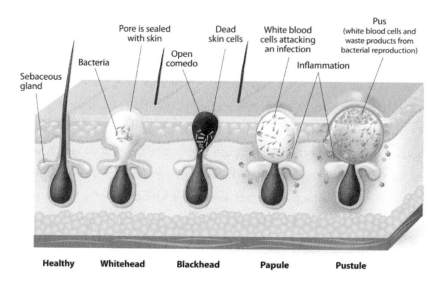

TYPES OF ACNE PIMPLES... ALONGSIDE INFECTED ONES

CONVENTIONAL
✳ ✳ ✳
ACNE TREATMENTS

Conventional methods for treating acne revolve around either killing *P. acnes* with prescription drugs or topicals like benzoyl peroxide or triclosan, or by slowing sebum production with anti-androgen drugs or Accutane.

Researchers have found that *P. acnes* is becoming increasingly resistant to some of the common antibiotics used to treat acne, like erythromycin and tetracycline and its derivatives, doxycycline and minocycline.

Several over-the-counter medications, specifically benzoyl peroxide and triclosan, are directly toxic to *P. acnes*. However, these medications don't penetrate to the base of the hair follicle where the problems start.

BENZOYL PEROXIDE, a strong bleach, is a sun sensitizer and should not be used over long periods of time.

TRICLOSAN is in a class of chemicals called chlorophenol, suspected of causing cancer in humans. To make matters even worse, triclosan degrades readily and in the presence of ultraviolet light converts to dioxin.

Dioxin exposure has been linked to cancer, birth defects, inability to maintain pregnancy, decreased fertility, reduced sperm counts, endometriosis, diabetes, learning disabilities, immune system suppression, lung problems, skin disorders, lowered testosterone levels and more.

CONVENTIONAL TREATMENTS TO DECREASE SEBUM PRODUCTION

№ 1 ORAL RETINOIDS: ISOTRETINOIN AND ACCUTANE

№ 2 TOPICAL RETINOIDS: RETIN-A AND ADAPALENE

№ 3 ANDROGEN INHIBITORS: SPIRONOLACTONE, CYPROTERONE AND BIRTH CONTROL PILLS

Everybody's acne has an individual profile, from origin to development to resolution. Hereditary factors play a big role in inflammatory acne, while puberty and concomitant raging testosterone is the major cause with teenage males. Adult acne, which affects 54% of the female population at some point, is also associated with hormonal fluctuations.

In some cases acne responds very well to relatively easy fixes. In other cases, it can be stubbornly resistant, and people may resort to the big guns like Accutane simply because they can't find anything else that works. And these days, some types of acne are resistant even to those treatments. So what is going on?

I believe another cause of skin problems like acne and other inflammatory disorders is microbial dysbiosis—an imbalance of microbial colonies in a community. For example, we're closer to understanding how the overuse of antibiotics can cause the gut flora that digest our food and fight off pathogens to be severely depleted, resulting in serious illnesses.

We set up conditions of skin microorganism imbalance every time we use topical antimicrobials. A case in point is triclosan. In small concentrations it kills *P. acnes* but not *Staph*, so you could trade a case of pimples for boils. In large concentrations it kills everything (including healthy skin cells), but since it also causes cancer and kills fish, it hardly seems worth it.

Most of the microflora on the skin, in addition to performing a wide range of other tasks, keep pathogens from invading.

Thus, the true answer to skin problems seems to lie in maintaining microbial balance. Rather than wiping out everything on the landscape, a more sensible approach might be to create an environment where the helpful microbes are free to create conditions in which pathogens do not thrive. It's all about the balance, or, as *Corynebacterium* would say, homeostasis.

The next chapter provides alternatives to conventional treatments by preventing acne at the source—effective ways to regulate sebum production without doing serious bodily harm.

SAFE ALTERNATIVES FOR TREATING ACNE

PREVENTION IS THE KEY TO FIGHTING ACNE OF ALL TYPES.
Pimples are born deep within the follicle. After sebum
and debris have clogged the pore, a plug, called a comedo,
forms. Whether infection develops into pimples depends on
your personal skin care habits—and even more on your
personal chemistry. Since all blemishes begin the same
way, everyone benefits from practices that prevent comedones from forming in the first place.

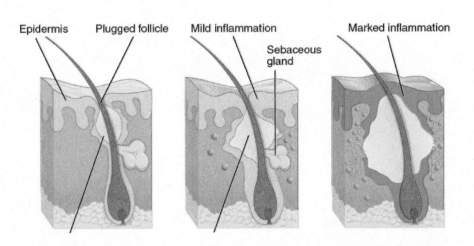

Epidermis   Plugged follicle   Mild inflammation   Marked inflammation

Sebaceous
gland

HISTORY OF A PIMPLE

CONTROLLING SEBUM
with VITAMIN B5

SEBUM production begins at puberty, coinciding with the first appearance of blemishes and acne. Sebum, a thick, waxy substance designed to lubricate the skin, combines with excess skin cells and clogs pores. When infection sets in, clogged pores become inflamed and develop into pimples. Excess sebum production is related to testosterone production, which explains why so many teenaged boys are plagued with acne. It makes sense that, just as acne starts with sebum, a safe and effective way to control it depends on finding a way to regulate sebum production.

Most sebum regulators have serious downsides, with Accutane (isotretinoin) topping the list. And with good reason—Accutane exacts a serious price, ranging from very dry skin to chronic bowel disorders like inflammatory bowel disease, Crohn's disease and ulcerative colitis to suicidal tendencies and even birth defects. Most of these side effects are chronic and remain even after the patient stops taking the drug. Available by prescription only, its use should be restricted to severe cases of acne that have not responded to other treatment protocols. If you've tried everything and are considering Accutane, I suggest you give the following little-known alternatives a try first.

VITAMIN B5 Like Accutane, vitamin B5 (aka pantothenic acid) works to control excess sebum production. Unlike Accutane, it does so without compromising sebaceous gland function. Instead it addresses the problem by increasing levels of Coenzyme-A (the body needs pantothenic acid to bio-synthesize Co-A), which in turn increases the body's ability to break down fats, including sebum. An excerpt from Dr. Leung's study in the *Journal of Orthomolecular Medicine* describes how effective pantothenic acid can be in clearing up even serious acne problems. For a more detailed account, read the complete study "A Stone that Kills Two Birds" at http://orthomolecular.org/library/jom/1997/pdf/1997-v12n02-p099.pdf.

THE EFFECT OF
* * *
PANTOTHENIC ACID ON ACNE VULGARIS

by DR. LIT-HUNG LEUNG

One hundred patients of Chinese descent were included in the study, 45 males and 55 females. The age ranged from 10 to 30, and with about 80% between 13 and 23. The severity of the disease process varied. They were given 10 grams of pantothenic acid a day in four divided doses. To enhance the effect, the patients were also asked to apply a cream consisting of 20% by weight of pantothenic acid to the affected area, four to six times a day. With this treatment regimen, the response is as prompt as it is impressive.

There is a noticeable decrease in sebum secretion on the face usually two to three days after initiation of therapy. The face becomes less oily.

After two weeks, existing lesions start to regress while the rate of eruption of new acne lesions begins to slow down.

In cases with moderate severity, the condition is normally in complete control in about eight weeks, with most of the lesions gone and new lesions only to erupt occasionally. In those patients with severe acne lesions, complete control may take months, sometimes up to six months or longer.

In some of these cases, in order to get a more immediate response, it may even be necessary to step up the dose to 15-20 grams a day. In any event, the improvement is normally a gradual and steady process, with perhaps minor interruptions by premenstrual flare or excessive intakes of oily food. With this form of treatment, another striking feature is the size of the facial skin pore. The pore size becomes noticeably smaller within one to two weeks, very often much sooner. Like sebum excretion, the pores will continue to shrink until the skin becomes much finer, giving the patient a much more beautiful skin.[1]

VITAMIN A DERIVATIVES

Topical retinoids like Retin-A (retinoic acid) may be prescribed for moderate-to-severe acne. Topical retinoids are an excellent treatment because they work on so many levels to ameliorate the condition.

Vitamin A derivatives are fat-soluble so they penetrate deep into the skin and into the sebaceous gland. Once there they bind to sebocyte receptors and help slow up sebum production.

RETINOIDS also bind to retinoic acid receptors, which govern age-repair processes like collagen production and breakdown. Retinoic acid receptors dictate how your skin sheds and renews itself, which not only decreases pore plugging, but also regulates the skin's natural enzymes and reduce inflammation.

RETIN-A is retinoic acid (aka tretinoin). It sometimes causes irritation and redness, discouraging people from sticking with it for the months that may be necessary to see improvement. Retinol is less harsh and may be a good alternative for people with sensitive skin. Since retinoids are the gold standard for acne care, it's a very good idea to find one you can use.

OTHER USEFUL VITAMINS

VITAMIN C is anti-inflammatory. Leukotrienes, the inflammatory chemical, are sometimes redirected towards the skin by bacteria like *P. acnes*, which they're sent to destroy, resulting in red and inflamed skin. Vitamin C can calm the immune system and inhibit inflammation.

VITAMIN E works best with vitamin C, as they complement each other's antioxidant activity. Vitamin E stabilizes oils secreted from the sebaceous gland and prevents them going rancid and hardening in the pore. Because it's an oil-soluble antioxidant, vitamin E also helps prevent damage to cell membranes. Perhaps its most important function is to help regulate levels of all-important retinol in the skin.

VITAMIN D3 Vitamin D has a number of benefits for acne treatment. It suppresses cell proliferation in the sebaceous glands and limits sebum production. Vitamin D3 is a major regulator of the expression of the antimicrobial peptide cathelicidin in epidermal keratinocytes.

OTHER NUTRIENTS

SOD When the body is subject to oxidative stress, it produces an enzyme called superoxide dismutase (SOD) to scavenge superoxide anions. Superoxide anions are highly destructive free radicals that destroy cell membranes and even DNA. When skin cells called keratinocytes are exposed to *P. acnes* they produce superoxide ions, and people who produce more SOD experience fewer and less intense breakouts. This forms the basis of a current theory: the skin's failure to produce sufficient superoxide dismutase is a major contributor to acne. If the skin does not produce sufficient SOD to dismutate the superoxide ions, excess superoxide ions kill skin cells and create inflammation.

MINERALS and TRACE MINERALS

ZINC GLUCONATE Zinc reduces the immune system's release of inflammatory chemicals at the earliest stages of acne. It is especially useful for preventing whiteheads and blackheads. Zinc gluoconate is the best oral supplement, and zinc oxide in sunscreen gets zinc to exactly where it's needed in the skin.

MINERALS LIKE SELENIUM, though needed in tiny amounts, are crucial to maintain proper antioxidant activity. Its lack is implicated in various skin problems as well as acne formation. Mineral deficiencies have become commonplace, with an estimated 90% of the population being mineral-deficient. This is a result of agribusiness depleting the soil of trace nutrients normally taken up by plants, which we then consume.

RELIEVING CONGESTION by EXFOLIATION

Another aspect of acne to consider is congestion, which we now know is how acne begins. The typical birth of a pimple brews below the surface, where excess sebum combines with dead cells to plug pores. The resulting comedones can remain in the blackhead stage, but if inflammation sets in expect pustules and pimples to follow.

AHAS AND OTHER PEELS attempt to clear out congestion, with hit-or-miss success. Unfortunately, purging skin of "excess oiliness and dirt" as instructed will not reach problems already well under way. In fact, too much exfoliation can dry and irritate skin—an open invitation to a bacterial invasion from the outside, thus exacerbating the breakout problem. Fortunately, one hydroxy acid can be used successfully—the beta hydroxy acid or salicylic acid.

SALICYLIC ACID concentrates at the surface of the pores and dissolves plugs that form there. This BHA dissolves protein from the outside in, and consistent use will prevent new open comedones from forming as well as further congestion of pores. Please note that in rare cases the FDA[2] warns of potentially severe allergic reactions to salicylic acid. Discontinue use and consult a physician if you experience symptoms including throat tightness, shortness of breath, wheezing, low blood pressure, fainting or collapse. If you develop hives or itching discontinue use.

RELIEVING CONGESTION
with LIPIDS

SEBUM in people prone to acne has been found to be deficient in linoleic acid—the omega-6-type essential fatty acid. Sebum deficient in linoleic acid is hard and sticky and clogs pores. The sebum looks greasy and has fewer protective and anti-inflammatory properties. I've had customers, particularly males, complain about the fact that their skins felt greasy rather than oily. I believe linoleic acid deficiency could account for skin that feels greasy, especially a few hours after cleansing. Altering the sebum lipid profile by applying topical oils keeps sebum lipids flowing and pores congestion free.

LINOLEIC ACID is also one of the key components of ceramides. Ceramides are composed of fatty acids and sphingosines and make up 50% of the stratum corneum.

THE STRATUM CORNEUM AND LIPIDS An intact stratum corneum (SC) is crucial to proper barrier function. The ability of the skin to both restrict water loss from the skin and prevent entry of pathogens depends on SC design, which consists of dead skin cells (keratinocytes) held together by lipids, arranged in a series of bilayers.

While the role of lipid interaction with bacteria to achieve protection is still poorly understood, we can identify three lipids that exhibit robust antibacterial activity: free fatty acids, glucosylceramides and sphingosines.

FREE FATTY ACIDS Triglycerides, the major component of sebum, are hydrolyzed by *P. acnes* to form free fatty acids. Free fatty acids like lauric acid and octadecanedioic acid orchestrate in harmony with other epidermal surface lipids to protect against pathogenic assault.

CERAMIDES An impaired water barrier function caused by decreased amounts of ceramides may be responsible for comedo formation. We suspect this is the case because barrier dysfunction is accompanied by hyperkeratosis of the follicular epithelium (thickening of the follicular walls due to increased quantity of dead skin cells).

SPHINGOSINE A ceramide is composed of sphingosine and a fatty acid, so a ceramide deficient skin barrier is also lacking sphingosine. Lipids, including sphingosines, control the survival of microorganisms on the SC.

the WONDERFUL WORLD of LIPIDS

We anticipate the emerging field of lipidomics to eventually shed light on intriguing dermatological diseases such as acne and atopic dermatitis that scientists currently do not associate with the epidermal surface lipids.

Topical ingredients that penetrate well and have the ability to dissolve compacted matter include salicylic acid, retinol and oils. Of those three, retinol and oils are excellent for dry, aging skins. And of those two, oils work best to alleviate dryness.

OIL & OIL-BLEND BENEFITS

№ 1   KEEPING PORES CLEAR

Oils penetrate the epidermal barrier and reach the source of the congestion. Omega-6 oils relieve congestion by promoting free flow of sebum in the pores.

№ 2   EXFOLIATION

Because oils dissolve oils, they can efficiently dissolve impacted matter in congested pores. And because they penetrate well, reaching far below the surface where congestion starts—considerably farther than conventional exfoliants that only scratch the surface, literally.

№ 3   KEEPING *P. ACNES* IN CHECK

Essential oils like tea tree oil are virtually as effective at killing *P. acnes* as benzoyl peroxide, with no downside.

№ 4   KEEPING THE BARRIER FUNCTION OPTIMAL

The stratum corneum requires near-constant replenishment as we get older. This is especially true during extreme weather, when skin is stripped of the oils designed to protect against bacterial attack—and keep skin soft and supple.

Science first exposed the falsehood of fat-free diets ("eating fats makes you fat"—it doesn't). Now it's time to embrace the concept that oil-free products can be as detrimental to our skins as fat-free diets are to our bodies.

The same can be said of the myth that oils cause the skin to break out. On the contrary, oils help keep your skin both youthful and blemish-free.

EVERYDAY
✳ ACNE-FIGHTING ✳
ROUTINES

SECTION 2 features routines to treat acne of different types. We'll provide an intimate look at adult acne, men's skin and acne vulgaris. Later, we'll explore conditions like rosacea, which is related to inflammation.

Mild acne can generally be cleared up by following all the topical treatment steps. More severe cases might benefit from internal supplementation as well.

Suggested supplements accompany the recommended topical treatments.

RESOURCES:

1. (http://orthomolecular.org/library/jom/1997/pdf/1997-v12n02-p099.pdf) "A Stone that Kills two Birds: How PantothenicAcid Unveils the Mysteries of Acne Vulgaris and Obesity," Lit-Hung Leung. M.D., Journal of Orthomolecular Medicine Vol.12, No.2, 1997

2. FDA: Topical Acne Products Can Cause Dangerous Side Effects

---

SAFE ALTERNATIVES FROM YOUR KITCHEN

MICROBIAL BALANCE IN THE GUT is a relatively new frontier and skin microbiotic balance is even newer. Scientists are studying how beneficial bacteria applied topically to the skin can work to interfere with the development of acne.

BENEFITS OF
* * *
TOPICAL PROBIOTICS

PROTECTIVE SHIELD Through a mechanism known as "bacterial interference," the body's immune system is distracted by harmless probiotic bacteria sitting on the skin's surface, doesn't invoke an inflammatory response to them, and misses other potential threats that might cause it to react. The result is less inflammation.

ANTIMICROBIAL DEFENSE We've learned that some microbes have bactericidal properties to aid in limiting pathogens. Probiotics as well as resident bacteria can produce antimicrobial peptides that benefit cutaneous immune responses and eliminate pathogens.[1]

CALMING EFFECT Other types of probiotics signal skin cells to arrest attack messages coming from the immune system.

STRENGTHENED SKIN BARRIER FUNCTION Very dry, damaged or acneic skin has reduced numbers of ceramides.

In a 2008 study[2], Dr. L Di Marzio and colleagues, for a limited-time period, applied a cream containing the probiotic *Streptococcus salivarius ssp. thermophilus* (*S. thermophilus*) to the skin of elderly Caucasian women.

In accordance with results of earlier experiments, the skin of the women who received the *S. thermophilus* cream showed increased skin ceramide level 1 over the control group. Their skin also showed increased hydration.

APPLE CIDER VINEGAR as a pH ADJUSTER

Normal skin is slightly acidic with a pH of 4 to 6.5. The microflora we have come to appreciate for the role they play in keeping skin healthy grow best at acidic pH levels, whereas *S. aureus*, the pathogen, prefers a neutral pH.

Shifts in the pH balance to alkaline can compromise skin's barrier function for up to 14 hours, the time it takes the skin to return to normal.

ACV as a FLAVONOID

A very recent study[3] shows that phloretin, a flavonoid found in apple cider vinegar, has significant anti-inflammatory and anti-acne properties.

GREEN TEA

ANOTHER FLAVONOID TO DRINK, TO WEAR—IT'S ALL GOOD

A two-part study in the December 2012 issue of the *Journal of Investigative Dermatology* showed that green tea helps to reduce sebum production. In the first part, the South Korean researchers applied cream containing epigallo-catechin gallate (EGCG) to rabbit ears and discovered that it reduced the size of sebaceous glands.

The second part of the test was conducted *in vitro* (petri dish) and involved the incubation of human sebocytes (sebum-producing cells) in insulin-like growth factor 1 (IGF-1) hormone. Several similar studies showed that IGF-1 increases sebocyte growth and also is one of the hormones linked to acne and oily skin.[4]

Researchers in stage two of the test added EGCG to the mix and subsequently found that IGF-1-induced cell growth and sebum production was significantly decreased, making the properties of EGCG ideal for treating acne. Further findings showed that an additional property of EGCG tended to suppress proinflammatory cytokines, a cause of systematic inflammation. Cytokines are cell-signaling molecules that communicate with the immune system.

Studies show acne-prone skin to be excessively sensitive to androgen hormones, causing an abnormally high production of sebum and skin cell growth.

The other significant cause of acne, as shown by leading-edge research, is inflammatory damage to sebum, which seems to trigger acne formation.

Studies show that green tea[5] can tackle both. The effect of androgens can be markedly reduced with green tea because EGCG blocks the conversion of testosterone to dihydrotestosterone (DHT) in the skin. Plus, EGCG has anti-inflammatory properties and, as such, helps protect against inflammation caused by UV rays or air pollution.

NEW PERSPECTIVES ON ACNE

TOPICAL APPLICATIONS

Even if you cut the claims made for topical green tea by half, they're still impressive. Read on for findings on applying a 2% green tea lotion to the skin:

REDUCES SEBUM PRODUCTION BY 70% by hindering conversion of testosterone to DHT in the skin.

HAS UVB PROTECTIVE PROPERTIES The high-powered antioxidants, polyphenols and catechins, in green tea offer some UVB protection. Sun protection can make a huge difference in treating acne, since UV exposure can exacerbate it by increasing inflammation via erythema.

REDUCES INFLAMMATORY RESPONSE in people with immune system dysfunction, which creates inflammatory acne. Again, it's thanks to the polyphenols and catechins, and something called epigallocatechin.

TURMERIC

Turmeric root contains curcuminoids, which have antioxidant and cancer-inhibiting properties. Many laboratory studies have identified a variety of molecules involved in inflammation that are inhibited by curcumin: phospholipase, lipooxygenase, cyclooxygenase-2, leukotrienes, prostaglandins, nitric oxide, collagenase, elastase and hyaluronidase.

We've covered acne causes and conventional and safe alternative treatment options, but key to fighting acne is learning the DOs and DON'Ts of PREVENTION.

PREVENTION IS KEY

Prevention is crucial to successfully fighting any type of acne. Pimples begin deep within the follicle. After sebum and debris clog the pore, a comedo forms. Infection may or may not develop into pimples; it's mostly a matter of personal chemistry. And since all blemishes begin the same way (via clogged pores and comedones), we all benefit knowing how to prevent comedones from forming initially. Read on for the dos and don'ts of prevention practices.

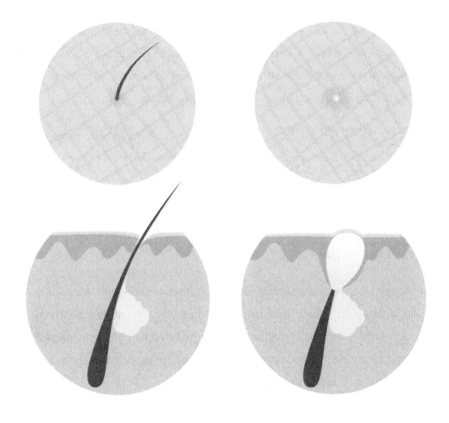

ACNE DEVELOPMENT

DO Wash your face now and again to get rid of excess grime. A gentle liquid soap with a pH around 4-5 is fine.

NEW PERSPECTIVES ON ACNE

DON'T Use soaps and cleansers that are too alkaline (high pH). They'll dry out your skin, disrupting barrier function that minimizes pathogenic assault. Avoid cleansers containing triclosan; it disrupts microbiota balance. Using too much triclosan can kill *P. acnes* without killing *Staphylococcus aureus*, resulting in boils instead of pimples.

DO Exfoliate with cleansers and masks containing lactic acid or sodium salicylate. Sodium salicylate is the salt of salicylic acid and has anti-inflammatory effects.

Salicylic acid can also be used, but the FDA has issued a warning about rare yet serious allergic reactions. If you develop extreme redness or a rash from an SA product, discontinue use immediately.

DON'T Exfoliate with scrubs containing sharp particles that cause microscopic tears in the skin and invite invasion from unfriendly microbes like *Staphylococcus aureus* and *Streptococcus pyogenes*.

DO Use toners that maintain a low pH on the skin's surface, around 3-4. Pathogens prefer high pH environments.

DON'T Use alcohol or other harsh toners that dry out your skin. They compromise the lipid barrier that protects from pathogenic attack.

DO Keep pores clear with oils high in linoleic and linolenic essential fatty acids. Linoleic acid-rich oils like safflower, sunflower, pumpkin and sesame seed are especially important for maintaining proper sebum flow.

DON'T Be oil-phobic. Oils dislodge the dried sebum and debris stuck in the pores—particularly oils in the omega-6 family, because oils dissolve oils.

DO Balance omega-6 with omega-3 (linolenic acid) oils in your topical oil blend. They inhibit production of prostaglandins, naturally occurring hormone-like substances that can increase inflammation. Omega-3 oils include flaxseed and chia seed; oils high in eicosapentaenoic acid (EPA), a valuable anti-inflammatory, can be found in fish, krill and some algae.

DON'T Use moisturizers containing wax or antimicrobial preservatives like parabens, phenoxyenthanol or sodium benzoate. Wax clogs pores and harsh antimicrobial preservatives are known skin irritants, probably because they exert microbial dysbiotic effects.

DO Use essential oils like tea tree oil. Studies show that tea tree oil helps control *P. acnes* populations as equally well as benzoyl peroxide, but without the side effects.

DON'T Use sulfur or clay more than two times a week. It dries the skin on the surface, causing further irritation and potentially leads to more breakouts. Don't try to dry out surface oil—by then it's too late!

DO Use a retin-based product. Vitamin A is the skin vitamin. It's so good you can think of the 'A' standing for 'age support' as well as 'acne combat.' On the acne-fighting front, it penetrates to sebaceous glands and reduces sebum production by binding to sebocyte receptors. Its anti-inflammatory effects keep *P. acnes* in check.

How carefully you choose your retinoid is key. Bear in mind that retinoic acid is the active ingredient that repairs photoaging and alleviates acne. Your skin can only use retinoids that are retinoic acid or, like retinol, can be converted to it—but retinol is not retinoic acid.

Retinol takes two steps to convert to retinoic acid (retinol → retinaldehyde → retinoic acid), so it's weaker than retinoic acid. If you opt to use straight-up retinoic acid, ask your dermatologist to help find the right prescription for you. Many people prefer over-the-counter retinol because it's generally less irritating, but that may be because the concentration is too low to do the job.

DO Look for a product with the following profile:

→ CONTAINS AN ENCAPSULATED VERSION OF RETINOL (PROTECTS AGAINST DEGRADATION)

→ CONTAINS AN EFFECTIVE CONCENTRATION OF RETINOL

→ DOES NOT CONTAIN RETINYL PALMITATE (TOO FAR REMOVED IN THE CONVERSION CHAIN)

DON'T Use benzoyl peroxide if you're an adult with acne. BP impedes new cell formation, and prolonged use photosensitizes skin, thus accelerating skin aging. Besides, neither antimicrobial topicals nor BP penetrates enough to disable *P. acnes.*

RESOURCES:

1. American Academy of Dermatology: "Could probiotics be the next big thing in acne and rosacea treatments?" SCHAUMBURG, Ill. (Feb. 3, 2014)

2. HealthyGutBugs.com: "Probiotics: The Best Anti-Aging Elixir for Your Skin?" March 13, 2014 By Jennifer Porteus

3. (http://www.ncbi.nlm.nih.gov/pubmed/26212527) "Evaluation of anti-acne properties of phloretin in vitro and in vivo," by Kum, H, Roh KB et.al., International Journal of Cosmetic Science, Feb, 2016

4. (http://www.acneeinstein.com/hormonal-acne/) Acne Einstein: "Hormonal Acne: How Hormones Affect The Skin," by Seppo Puusa

5. Natural News: "Green tea boosts your brain power, especially your working memory" 7/15/2015

ROSACEA: IT'S NOT ACNE

ROSACEA AND ACNE SHARE AN ORIGIN IN INFLAMMATION, BUT THE CLINICAL MANIFESTATIONS ARE QUITE DIFFERENT. Rosacea and acne should never be treated the same way, as there's a good chance you will simply irritate the skin, increase inflammation and exacerbate the problem.

~~~~~~

✳ IDENTIFYING ROSACEA ✳
DESCRIPTION and SYMPTOMS

Rosacea is increasingly more common and gaining in numbers, but interpreting the data on who develops it is difficult. Data suggests that rosacea is slightly more likely to occur in women, but men are more likely to get severe cases, involving rhinophyma, for example. Speaking at the anecdotal level as a skin care practitioner, I see countless cases of rosacea that go undiagnosed and untreated, especially among men. I suspect conventional data underreports rosacea among men, and data regarding men experiencing more severe symptoms than women adds weight to my theory. In general, women will get the 'red alert' long before the Rudolf-the-Red-Nosed-Reindeer stage, and seek some relief. They're ready to try almost anything and not about to wait for the situation to get out of control.

Rosacea tends to show up around ages 30 to 50 and affect fair-skinned people of Celtic or Nordic heritage to the extent that it is called the Celtic curse.
However anyone can get this disease, including children and people of color.
One cross-ethnic common denominator is that rosacea sufferers often bat-
tled acne when they were younger.

Symptoms vary to such a degree that four separate subtypes have been identified. Rosacea sufferers may have multiple subtypes simultaneously.

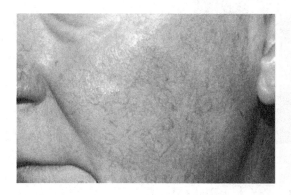

SUBTYPE 1:
Numerous dilated
capillaries
or spider veins

ROSACEA SUBTYPE 1:
FACIAL REDNESS and FLUSHING

The symptoms most commonly associated with rosacea:

→ FACIAL FLUSHING THAT CAN BECOME PERMANENT
  REDNESS, GENERALLY IN THE CENTER OF THE FACE

→ DILATED BLOOD VESSELS (SPIDER VEINS)

→ SWOLLEN, HOT TO THE TOUCH, FEELINGS OF STINGING
  OR BURNING

→ DRY, ROUGH, SCALY, SENSITIVE

A tendency to flush more easily than others, and the flush takes longer to sub-side. Flushing in heat or when exercising is normal, but one way to identify rosacea is the length of time it takes for dilated capillaries to shrink. Flushing recedes in 1-2 minutes in normal skin; with rosacea a flush may last for hours. At some point the vascular system may be so compromised the skin becomes permanently red.

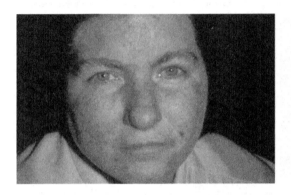

SUBTYPE 2:
Extensive rash-like
eruptions on cheeks
and forehead

ROSACEA SUBTYPE 2: ACNE-LIKE BREAKOUTS

These symptoms create the confusion between acne and rosacea. In fact, it's still sometimes called "acne rosacea."

→ BREAKOUTS LOOK LIKE ACNE PUSTULES AT FIRST GLANCE, BUT ARE GENERALLY MORE RASH-LIKE, COVERING GREATER AREA WITH SMALL, UNPRODUCTIVE BUMPS—NOT FILLED WITH PUS

→ RASHES CAN COME AND GO, USUALLY ACCOMPANIED BY REDNESS AND FEELINGS OF STINGING AND BURNING

→ VISIBLE SPIDER VEINS

→ RAISED PATCHES OF SKIN CALLED PLAQUES

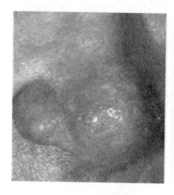

SUBTYPE 3:
An example of rhinophyma

ROSACEA SUBTYPE 3: THICKENING SKIN

This is rare and usually occurs as a later stage of rosacea development. People with this type of rosacea are often unfairly identified as alcoholic. W. C. Fields was lucky enough to transform his skin disease into economic gold. Most outcomes are not so positive. Symptoms are:

→ BUMPY SKIN TEXTURE

→ SKIN BEGINS TO THICKEN, ESPECIALLY PREVALENT ON THE NOSE, CALLED RHINOPHYMA

→ SKIN MAY THICKEN ON THE CHIN, FOREHEAD, CHEEKS AND EARS

→ VISIBLE BROKEN BLOOD VESSELS APPEAR

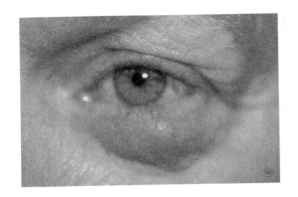

SUBTYPE 4:
OCULAR ROSACEA

About 50% of people with other types of rosacea also suffer from ocular rosacea; some people have ocular rosacea exclusively and no symptoms elsewhere.

→ EYES WATER EASILY AND MAY APPEAR BLOODSHOT

→ EYES BURN OR STING AND OFTEN FEEL GRITTY, LIKE THEY HAVE SAND IN THEM

→ DRY AND ITCHY, SENSITIVE TO LIGHT

→ BLURRED VISION

→ BLEPHARITIS OR INFLAMMATION OF THE EYELIDS, OR EYELID CYSTS

NEW PERSPECTIVES ON ACNE

ROSACEA PATHOGENESIS

We know rosacea is inflammatory in origin and characterized by facial or ocular inflammation involving both the vascular and connective tissue. Beyond that past discussions have been limited to identifying the diverse factors that might exacerbate or improve the disease. Exciting developments in recent research have begun to shed more light on the source of the inflammation.

The pathophysiology of rosacea involves a complex interaction of different factors and pathways leading to a chronic inflammatory and vascular response. Researchers like Dr. Richard L. Gallo have made great strides in elucidating the molecular mechanisms causing the disease. It's a fascinating journey that begins with antimicrobial peptides[1].

Antimicrobial peptides (AMPs) are part of the innate immune system. Most AMPs are members of the defensin and cathelicidin peptide families. Cathelicidin peptides, produced by keratinocytes (skin cells), can destroy bacteria, viruses and yeast. The innate immune system or pattern recognition system includes Toll-like receptor (TLR) families. Triggering the innate immune system normally leads to a controlled increase in cytokines and AMPs like cathelicidins in the skin.

Triggers that include UV exposure, altered hormonal balance, microbes and chemical or physical trauma can increase levels of TLR-2, and activation of TLR-2 induces an increase in cathelicidin and kallikrein 5 (KLK5). Cathelicidin peptides are processed by serine proteases of the kallikrein 5 (KLK5) family. Interestingly, the entire epidermis of rosacea-type skin shows increased expression of KLK5 and subsequently high protease activity. The serine protease activity results in proinflammatory forms of the antimicrobial peptide, such as LL-37. Peptides like LL-37 go on to cause the inflammatory skin response.

Rosacea patients also have greatly elevated levels of enzymes called stratum corneum tryptic enzymes (SCTE). These enzymes turn the precursor cathelicidin into the abnormal, disease-causing peptides.

In what Dr. Gallo calls a "trifecta of unfortunate factors," these vasoactive and proinflammatory peptides promote the changes in tissue observed in rosacea. Similar tissue changes have also been observed in psoriasis patients.

ACCORDING TO DR. GALLO:

"Too much SCTE and too much cathelicidin lead to the abnormal peptides that cause the symptoms of this disease. Antibiotics tend to alleviate the symptoms of rosacea in patients because some of them work to inhibit these enzymes. Our findings may modify the therapeutic approach to treating rosacea, since bacteria aren't the right target."

The original study and research was undertaken by Richard L. Gallo, M.D., Ph.D., of the University of California in San Diego, and colleagues with support from the National Institutes of Health and the National Rosacea Society.

ROSACEA TRIGGERS

Microbes and environmental changes, such as sun, heat and UV exposure are sensed by pattern recognition molecules (Toll-like receptors or TLRs). The innate immune system cathelicidin response is enhanced by cytokine, reactive oxygen species (ROS), antimicrobial peptides and proteases. With rosacea, the abnormalities in the innate immune system create an inflammatory response leading to tissue changes.

We can correlate the severity of symptoms with the number and degree of intensity of the stressors on the immune system to some extent, but an individual's susceptibility to one or more contributing factors handicaps diagnosing treatments on anything other than a case-by-case basis. Nonetheless outlining a treatment protocol starts with pinpointing the major triggers to inflammation and subsequent tissue changes.

EMFs — MODERN ROSACEA TRIGGER?

A potential threat to skin integrity has hit the scene: hypersensitivity to electric and magnetic fields (EMFs), with first cases reported nearly 20 years ago.

Those reports indicated cutaneous problems as well as symptoms from internal organs, like the heart, in people exposed to video display terminals.

Symptoms such as itching, heat sensation, pain, erythema, papules and pustules appeared to come from the phenomenon 'screen dermatitis'.

To researchers like Patrick Levallois we're far from understanding this phenomenon since those first reports. He concludes[1] that while "the literature on the subject is still very limited... it appears that the so-called hypersensitivity to environmental electric and magnetic fields is an unclear health problem whose nature has yet to be determined."[2]

Literature may be thin, but countering arguments can be found in the work of Dr. Olle Johansson, The Experimental Dermatology Unit, Department of Neuroscience, Karolinska Institute, Stockholm. His evidence-based case links EMF exposure to public health problems; his conclusions are crystal clear.

№ 1 "Measurable physiological changes (mast cells increases, for example) that are bedrock indicators of allergic response and inflammatory conditions are stimulated by EMF exposures."[3]

№ 2 "Chronic exposure to such factors that increase allergic and inflammatory responses on a continuing basis may be harmful to health."

№ 3 "It is possible that chronic provocation by exposure to EMF can lead to immune dysfunction, chronic allergic responses, inflammatory responses and ill health if they occur on a continuing basis over time."[4]

ADD EMFs to your TRIGGER LIST?

If you notice that symptoms like redness, burning, itching or stinging of skin occur when EMF exposure is high (for example, while talking on your cell phone), consider limiting your EMF exposure.

LIMIT EMF EXPOSURE

№ 1 Unplug things at night if you can; keep what must stay plugged in, out of your sleeping space.

№ 2 Spend less time at the computer; limit use of wireless devices.

№ 3 Limit cell phone use; use a landline instead.

№ 4 Don't carry your cell phone in your pocket. Turn it off more often.

№ 5 Avoid halogen, fluorescent tube and energy-efficient compact fluorescent lighting. All have intense EMF emissions.

UV EXPOSURE AND HEAT

UV exposure and heat cause flushing responses that result in prolonged redness and swelling via a number of mechanisms.

EPIDERMAL KERATINOCYTES are a major source of vascular endothelial growth factor (VEGF) and fibroblast growth factor 2 (FGF2). UVB rays increase secretion of both, increasing vascularization of skin, and swelling.

UVB AND UVA IRRADIATION also produce reactive oxygen species (ROS) causing vascular and dermal matrix damage by stimulating enzymes that break down collagen in the dermal matrix may permit leakage and accumulation of inflammatory mediators and prolonged retention of inflammatory cells.

UVB TRIGGERS ACTIVATION OF VITAMIN D3,[1] which directly induces the expression of cathelicidin.

MITES

The mite *Demodex folliculorum* lives within sebaceous follicles and has long been suspected of contributing to rosacea, since rosacea sufferers host about 50% more of the microorganisms than non-affected people.

LACEY ET AL isolated *Bacillus oleronius* from *D. folliculorum* and identified the antigens reacting to sera from rosacea individuals but not from control individuals.

The extracts of the *B. oleronius* stimulate proliferation of mononuclear cells from patients with rosacea, suggesting that a) rosacea individuals are exposed to the *B. oleronius* molecules, and b) *B. oleronius* from *D. folliculorum* induces inflammatory responses in rosacea.[2]

HEAT SHOCK PROTEINS (HSP) AND A LIPOPROTEIN were identified in the antigenic molecules of *B. oleronius*. HSP and lipoproteins from microbes are also known to be a stimulant for Toll-like receptors (TLRs).

Still to be investigated: whether these *B. oleronius* molecules evoke the innate immune reaction, or if rosacea is caused by adaptive immune reaction against *B. oleronius* and *D. folliculorum*.

CHITIN released from *Demodex* mites possibly triggers TLR2 activation and subsequent protease activity in the skin of rosacea patients.

ROSACEA TREATMENTS

UV EXPOSURE

Many people with rosacea do not tolerate sun well and are advised to limit their sun exposure. Since we all like at least some sun, the following suggestions will help boost your tolerance.

ZINC OXIDE SUNSCREEN is essential for rosacea-prone people. Because sun damage continues after the sun is no longer directly on your skin and because zinc oxide is a wonderful anti-inflammatory, add zinc oxide sunscreen to your nightly routine.

VITAMIN D3 is something everyone needs, but since vitamin D3 stimulates cathelicidn expression, apply sunblock to the areas where rosacea is a problem. Fortunately, you'll get enough vitamin D3 synthesis by exposing the rest of your body. Wait a bit before you shower, because vitamin D takes a while to synthesize from the oils on your skin.

ANTIOXIDANT SUPPLEMENTS should be taken daily, notably astaxanthin and lycopene. These antioxidants from the carotenoid family will increase your tolerance to the sun.

RETINOIDS help with inflammation by reducing signals that trigger cathelicidin production that blocks TLR-2 activity. Use a retinol or retinoid product nightly. **Be hypervigilant about sun protection if you use a retinoid product**.

TOPICAL ANTIOXIDANTS C AND E help control inflammation by neutralizing free radicals. Apply a topical antioxidant serum at night to accomplish two things: 1) The antioxidants will help arrest DNA damage to skin cells caused by chemiexcitation; and 2) you'll build up a reservoir of vitamin C that will help boost sun protection the next day. Vitamin C, once applied, does not wash off, and studies show it continues to work three days later. Take internally as well.

SUPPLEMENTS TO ADD

INTERNAL AND EXTERNAL

→ VITAMIN C with bioflavonoids, 500mg / 2 x a day

→ VITAMIN E, 400IU / 1 x a day

→ NIACINAMIDE (VITAMIN B3), 500mg / 1 x a day

→ ANTIOXIDANTS ASTAXANTHIN &/or LYCOPENE / 1 x a day

Look for these supplements in topical serums as well as taking them internally.

INTERNAL

→ CURCUMIN, 500 mgs 1 x a day

→ OMEGA-3 EFAs, 1-2 tbsps fish oil daily
The EPA type found in fish and krill oil. Eicosapentaenoic acid (EPA) can be found in some algae oils as well.

→ GREEN TEA EXTRACT
Look for the compound epigallocatechin gallate (ECGC)

the MICROORGANISM CONNECTION

Often people who suffered from acne as youngsters exhibit rosacea symptoms at later stages in life. While this has not been well explored to date, it is an interesting connection. *Demodex folliculorum* feed on sebum and are more prevalent following puberty, preferring to colonize sebaceous areas of the face.

Demodex mites may also feed on epithelial cells lining the pilosebaceous unit, or even on organisms (such as *P. acnes*) that inhabit the same space. Thus, over-production of sebum and over-colonization of *P. acnes* would lead to an exploding population of *D. folliculorum*. Even when acne is under control it might leave behind an exaggerated population of *Demodex* mites. While it's unclear whether rosacea results from an innate immune reaction from *B. oleronius* molecules or is caused by adaptive immune reaction against *B. oleronius* and *D. folliculorum*, the acne connection suggests that rosacea might be an artifact of adolescent acne. Only if mites are part of your overall acne picture could we consider miticidal treatments for rosacea—and acne.

MITICIDAL FACIAL SCRUB/MASK

→ GREEN MUNG BEAN, coarsely ground, 50g

→ NEEM LEAF, finely sieved powder, 50g

→ WHITE SANDALWOOD, finely sieved powder, 50g

GENTLE SCRUB Mix ingredients together; use a small handful with a bit of water to make a paste. Use as a facial scrub, gently rubbing over the affected area to exfoliate and remove the mites. You may also use this to control blepharitis; use in the same way, but apply very gently between the lashes with a cotton swab, then rinse.

MASK If area is too sensitive or irritated, apply paste over affected areas for 15-20 minutes, then remove with water. Gentle enough to use nightly.

TEA TREE OIL

Tea tree oil is an excellent miticide to use as soap or face wash daily. As well as commercial products, you may also make an oil blend with up to 25% tea tree oil. Purportedly the concentration of tea tree oil needs to be 50% to be effective, but this is very strong and will burn. I recommend using a 25% tea tree oil solution with 25% neem oil, a good miticide that is less irritating. If you have blepharitis and use this blend to kill eyelash mites, apply a tiny amount with a cotton swab, careful not to let it get in your eyes—it will sting.

MITICIDE OIL RECIPE

→ JOJOBA, SAFFLOWER OR SUNFLOWER OIL, 25 ml

→ TEA TREE OIL, 25 ml

→ SEA BUCKTHORN OIL, 25 ml

→ NEEM OIL, 25 ml

Mix ingredients together. Store in a cool place. Shake well before using. Mites come out at night to mate when it's dark, so it's best to apply a tiny amount to affected areas before bedtime. If you have an infestation, you may feel some perturbation from the critters encountering and reacting to the oil.

PROBIOTICS

The rosacea-type immune system response to invading microorganisms creates inflammation resulting in the redness and bumps characteristic of the disease. Here's how topically applied probiotics can help:

"BACTERIAL INTERFERENCE" Probiotics prevent skin cells from seeing the presence of "bad" bacteria and invoking an immune system response.

ANTIMICROBIAL PEPTIDES secreted by some probiotics can help keep pathogens under control.

A CALMING EFFECT is exerted by some probiotics when placed in contact with skin cells, thus averting the inflammatory response reaction.

YOGURT, OATMEAL & TURMERIC CLEANSER/MASK

→ WHOLE MILK YOGURT, 1-2 cups

→ GROUND OATMEAL, ¼ cup

→ TURMERIC, ½ tsp

Grind oatmeal in a blender to make a fine powder. Mix with yogurt and turmeric to make a paste. Store in a covered glass container. Keep refrigerated.

As a cleanser, take ½ tsp of the paste and gently apply all over face; rinse with warm water. To use as a mask, apply the same amount and leave on for 10-15 minutes; rinse with warm water.

Plain yogurt can also be used as a moisturizer. Apply a very thin layer, just enough so it disappears into the skin, about ⅛ tsp. Let dry. Cover with sunscreen in the morning, and at night follow the yogurt layer with serums as usual.

ANTI-INFLAMMATORIES

GREEN TEA

Green tea is a wonderfully soothing way to treat rosacea flare-ups.

ANTI-INFLAMMATORY properties calm skin.

UVB PROTECTIVE properties reduce secretion of the factors: vascular endothelial growth factor (VEGF) and fibroblast growth factor 2 (FGF2), which increase vascularization of the skin and swelling.

LIMIT FREE RADICAL DAMAGE with polyphenols and catechins.

GREEN TEA MIST

Steep 4-5 green tea bags in 1 qt water. Let cool. Pour into a mist bottle and spray it on morning and night as part of your routine. Mist any time your skin needs calming. It's indispensable whenever you're out of doors.

NIACINAMIDE & ZINC

Both of these powerful anti-inflammatories are being studied for their efficacy in treating inflammatory diseases like acne vulgaris.

NIACINAMIDE AND ZINC LOTION

At night, combine a pea-sized amount of serum containing niacinamde with a similar amount of your zinc oxide sunscreen in the palm of your hand. Apply as the final step of your nightly routine.

RESOURCES:

1. PubMed.gov: J Immunol. 2004 Sep 1;173(5):2909-12. *Cutting edge: 1,25-dihydroxyvitamin D3 is a direct inducer of antimicrobial peptide gene expression.*

2. Environ Health Perspect. 2002 Aug; 110(Suppl 4): 613–618 *Hypersensitivity of human subjects to environmental electric and magnetic field exposure: a review of the literature, by Patrick Levallois*

3. PubMed.gov: Med Hypotheses. 2000 Apr;54(4):663-71. *A theoretical model based upon mast cells and histamine to explain the recently proclaimed sensitivity to electric and/or magnetic fields in humans. Gangi S, Johansson O.*

4. (http://www.bioinitiative.org/report/wp-content/uploads/pdfs/sec08_2007_Evidence_%20Effects_%20Immune_System.pdf) *BioInitiative 2012, Section 8. Evidence for Effects on the Immune System, by Olle Johansson, PhD*

MEN'S SKIN

THANKS TO TESTOSTERONE, MEN'S SKIN DIFFERS FROM
WOMEN'S SKIN IN FOUR SIGNIFICANT WAYS:

№ 1 HIGHER CONCENTRATION OF BLOOD VESSELS
Men have a larger number and a higher concentration
of blood vessels, especially on the cheekbones

№ 2 RICHER HYDROLIPIDIC FILM
The sebaceous glands, which are responsible for
sebum production, are larger, more numerous and more
active in men than in women

№ 3 THICKER SKIN
Men's skin is about 25% thicker than women's skin

№ 4 MORE FACIAL HAIR
Testosterone stimulates the growth of facial hair

All of these differences help create the skin conditions men experience: razor bumps, blemishes and
breakouts into adulthood, and excessive redness.
As you've probably guessed, treating them requires
routines and products developed for men.

MEN AND ACNE

All acne, whether adult or teenage acne (acne vulgaris), starts when excess sebum clogs pores. This means acne starts deep down in the follicle, below the reach of anti-acne cleansers, masks and lotions. And because men's sebaceous glands exceed women's sebaceous glands in both number and activity, it is especially important to prevent sebum from clogging pores.

THE OIL CONUNDRUM

Men are often advised to use a moisturizer, since dry skin can aggravate inflammation and set the stage for future breakouts. However, not any moisturizer will do. Creams and lotions containing wax and oil-free moisturizers can clog pores and make acne worse. Unfortunately the mistaken equation "oils = oily skin = breakouts" still prevails in many circles. Actually skin needs oil, particularly oils high in omega 3s and 6s, to unclog pores. Using oils to moisturize is even more important if your skin produces sebum low in linoleic acid, the omega-6-type EFA. This EFA-deficient type of sebum is thick and sticky and readily clogs pores.

A common complaint from men with linoleic acid-deficient sebum is that their skin feels greasy instead of oily. Fortunately that greasy feeling can be easily remedied with use of an oil blend high in linoleic acid-rich oils, like safflower or sunflower oil. Another advantage of oils is that they breach barricades put up by facial hair and beard stubble far more effectively than lotions. Best of all, because oils dissolve oils, they break up congestion and prevent acne formation at the source. A big plus.

MEN'S SKIN MICROBIOME

Men's skin plays host to a variety of resident microbes like *Staphylococcus epidermidis* and *Propionibacterium acnes*. Transient microbial populations arising from the environment are also present and may persist for hours or days. These microbes are usually commensal, that is, not harmful and perhaps providing benefit to the host.

With good hygiene and as long as normal resident flora, immune responses and skin barrier functions are intact, both resident and transient microbes are not pathogenic. However, balance disruption can give resident and/or transient bacterial populations the opportunity to colonize, proliferate and cause disease.

One such disruption happens at puberty. Prior to puberty no sebum is produced, and *P. acnes*, which feeds on sebum, is rare. With the onset of puberty, sebaceous glands go into overdrive for both sexes, but the cells in a man's sebaceous glands have more positive receptors for androgens, so they'll produce more sebum going forward. Excess sebum production revs up the whole cycle—it invites over-colonization by *P. acnes*, which kicks off immune system responses that create inflammation and lead eventually to acne formation.

Teenage boys frequently suffer inflammatory or cystic acne. Young men with this type of acne should be under the care of a dermatologist, as it can be a very complicated picture with a bleak outlook of years and years of treatment if not handled properly.

Adult males may continue to have acne into their 30s and 40s, even after the puberty storm has settled, simply because they continue to produce more sebum. More facial hair also makes a difference. Hairy moist underarms lie a short distance from smooth dry forearms, but they have distinctly different resident microbial communities. Sweating creates an even more welcoming environment for pathogens. An inhospitable environment for microbial growth is skin that is cool, dry and acidic.

NEW PERSPECTIVES ON ACNE

DOS & DON'TS

* * *

TO HELP BREAK THE BREAKOUT CYCLE

DO Wash your face once or twice a day to rid skin of excess grime. Use a gentle liquid soap with a pH around 4-5.

DON'T Use soaps and cleansers that are too alkaline (high pH). They'll dry out skin, disrupting barrier function that works to minimize pathogenic assault.

DO Use toners that maintain a low pH (around 3-4) on the skin's surface. *Strep* and *Staph* pathogens prefer high pH environments. A splash of apple cider vinegar after cleansing or shaving will restore proper pH balance.

DON'T Use alcohol or other harsh toners that dry out your skin. You'll only compromise the lipid barrier that protects you from pathogenic attack.

DO Use moisturizers and cleansers that contain probiotics and few preservatives. In a pinch, yogurt makes a great cleanser and a decent moisturizer.

DON'T Use cleansers and moisturizers containing antimicrobials like parabens, triclosan and sodium benzoate. Cleansers containing triclosan or other antimicrobials will disrupt microbial balance. If you use too much triclosan and kill *P. acnes* without killing *Staphylococcus aureus*, you may even end up with boils instead of pimples. Don't use benzoyl peroxide. In the short term, this antimicrobial will kill *P. acnes*, but long-term side effects include sun sensitivity and accelerated aging.

DO Prevent sebum build-up in pores with oils high in linoleic and linolenic essential fatty acids. Linoleic acids, the omega 6s, are especially important for maintaining proper sebum flow. Your topical oil blend should also contain omega-3 (linolenic acid) oils in the proper balance.

Omega-3 oils, including flaxseed and chia seed, inhibit production of prostaglandins, naturally occurring hormone-like substances that can increase inflammation. Oils high in eicosapentaenoic acid (EPA) are valuable for anti-inflammatory effects and can be found in fish oil, krill oil and some algae oils.

DON'T Use "oil-free" as a reason to buy your daily moisturizer. Look instead for moisturizers that contain anti-acne agents like salicylic acid.

DO Find the vitamin A derivative (retinoid or retinol) right for your skin. Vitamin A is the skin vitamin that combats acne and repairs wrinkles. It is the essential ingredient in keeping skin clear and youthful.

DON'T Make choices based on misinformation about retinol/retinoids and how they work. Most retinol products simply do not have a high enough concentration of retinol to be effective. With over-the-counter products, look for high concentrations of retinol or retinaldehyde, and if they don't do the trick, check with a dermatologist about getting a prescription retinoid. Retinoids do work, so shop around to find the one that works for you.

DO Exfoliate with cleansers and masks containing lactic acid and sodium salicylate. Sodium salicylate is the salt of salicylic acid and has anti-inflammatory effects.

You may also use salicylic acid as long as you are not allergic. SA is a beta hydroxy acid that eats protein from the outside in and helps unclog pores.

However, do be aware of the warning issued by the FDA[1]. In rare cases SA can cause a severe allergic reaction. If you experience swelling, excessive redness or a rash using a mask or cleanser containing SA discontinue its use immediately.

DON'T Exfoliate with scrubs that contain sharp particles. These particles can cause microscopic tears in the skin, inviting invasions from unfriendly microbes like *Staphylococcus aureus* and *Streptococcus pyogenes*.

DO TAKE YOUR VITAMINS Some vitamins must be taken internally only, some topically only, and some may be taken both ways.

VITAMINS

VITAMIN B5 (or pantothenic acid) tops the list for men. The body draws from the available pool of B5 to not only make hormones, but also to make Coenzyme-A, which breaks down fats and sebum. During times of peak hormonal activity like puberty, the body's top priority is generating hormones, often leaving nothing left over for sebum and fat breakdown. The result: so many teenage boys with acne.

Vitamin B5 can be taken internally and applied topically. For mild adult acne, the topical treatment is often enough, but teenagers and adults with moderate to severe acne can take up to 10,000-20,000 mgs daily.

VITAMIN B3 Anti-inflammatory. Apply topically and take internally.

VITAMIN D3 Regulates sebaceous gland activity and sebum production, decreases overactive cell turnover rate to help keep pores clear. Take internally only.

VITAMIN C Anti-inflammatory that builds up capillary linings.

VITAMIN E Partnered with vitamin C, they support each other's antioxidant function. Both can and should be taken internally and applied topically.

ADDITIONAL SUPPLEMENTS

OMEGA-3 essential fatty acids, especially fish or algae oil high in EPA, (eicosapentaenoic acid): Anti-inflammatory. Can be taken internally and applied topically.

ZINC Reduces sebum and anti-inflammatory. Take internally as zinc gluconate. Take topically as zinc oxide in your sunscreen.

MINERALS AND TRACE MINERALS Find a mineral supplement that contains a full spectrum of minerals, including trace minerals.

PROBIOTICS Rebalances skin microbiome. Take internally and apply topically, for example by using yogurt in a mask.

DON'T TAKE TOO MANY SUPPLEMENTS especially oil-soluble vitamins like vitamin A.

SHAVING and the BEARD MICROBIOME

To shave or not to shave became the question recently when a story about beards containing poop went viral (or do we mean virile?). Apparently a microbiologist found some enteric bacteria in a few beard swabs sent to him by a television "news" program, and the ensuing announcement that beards were full of it got everyone talking.

Of course, the story offers endless opportunities to speculate imaginatively on how bacteria found in feces ended up on beard hair, but the real answer is less salaciously thrilling—unless you are a microbiologist of course.

Members of *Enterobacteriaceae* live in the gut and are certainly in feces. But most are commensal, and many bacteria, for example *S. epidermidis* and *P. acnes*, reside in both the skin and the gut. The real truth? Shit happens. It's happening all over us, inside and out, all the time, and we are beholden to our hardworking microbes for making it happen.

Nevertheless, beards probably do contain more bacteria than most places, if only because sebaceous glands on the face are larger than those on the head. Microbes may feast on the oil near the base of the hair duct, but it has not been established that beards carry more *P. acnes*. This should come as no surprise as its favorite habitat is deep in the sebaceous glands, far away from the skin's surface.

While acne and beards don't go together, eczema can be a problem, particularly if some soap remains after a beard washing.

Also, spicy or acidic foods trapped in beards can cause contact dermatitis. If you're looking for an ick factor I suggest you start there.

SHAVING

Suppose all this talk of beard bacteria has made you want to reach for the razor. This can also cause problems, by way of razor bumps or ingrown hairs, officially known as *psuedofolliculitis barbae*. They happen after you shave, as strands of hair curl back on themselves and grow into the skin. The result can be irritation, sometimes extreme, pimples and even scarring.

HELP to PREVENT RAZOR BUMPS

DO Exfoliate the skin with a cleanser containing salicylic acid.

DON'T Use glycolic acid—it does not have the same unclogging effect as SA, and it may cause irritation. Glycolic acid can also cause hyperpigmentation problems, particularly with African and Asian skin. Lactic acid is okay.

DO Rinse off the cleanser with warm water and keep your face moistened for the shave. This softens the coarse hair.

DON'T Rinse with cold water.

DO Lather up with a moisturizing shaving cream or gel.

DON'T Use plain soap, it is too alkaline

DO Shave in the direction of hair growth, using the fewest razor strokes possible.

DON'T Stretch the skin.

DO After shaving use an oil blend to make sure pores don't get clogged.

DON'T Use alcohol, which dries the skin and can cause irritation.

STAGES OF REDNESS

You may have noticed how many men appear to have permanently red faces. This makes sense, since men have a higher concentration of blood vessels, especially on the cheekbones.

When the skin's vessels dilate quickly, redness appears on the surface of the face, creating a flush. With normal skin the vessels quickly shrink, but with redness-prone and sensitive skins, the phenomenon may worsen and the vessels become more and more dilated and more visible. Eventually the redness becomes permanent. The stages of redness are very similar to rosacea:

HEAT Skin starts feeling hot, flushed and red intermittently. The sensations may come on without warning.

REDNESS becomes more persistent over time. Diffuse but permanent redness is called erythrosis and is most commonly located on the cheeks.

ROSACEA SYMPTOMS like red spots, often with whiteheads, can occur.

REDNESS FACTORS

UV EXPOSURE / HEAT cause the skin's microcirculation to speed up.

STRESS, either emotional or physical (vigorous exercise), causes flushing.

SKIN AGING After 25, the skin becomes increasingly sensitive to redness.

ROSACEA CONNECTION

The redness may be the first sign of developing rosacea, since the cause of all types of redness is hyper-reactivity of the skin's vessels. This hyper-reactivity is related to immune system responses that create cathelicidins of the proinflammatory and vasoactive type, which results in rosacea. Similar to rosacea, heredity plays a role in redness, especially in people with vasoreactive skin, a skin characteristic that can be familial.

Unlike most disorders, rosacea tends to affect men and women somewhat differently. Interestingly, redness, proliferation of the sebaceous glands and swelling of the skin on the nose (a condition known as rhinophyma found in extreme cases of rosacea) is only seen in males. In fact, 21% of men surveyed reported swelling of the nose associated with advanced rosacea, versus 8% of women. Women with rosacea are more likely to experience symptoms on the cheeks and chin.

NEUTRALIZING REDNESS in SENSITIVE SKIN

Forestalling later and more serious rosacea-related problems is best accomplished by nipping redness in the bud. Especially for men, treating early symptoms is by far the best way to avoid any really troublesome symptoms down the road. The other good argument for early treatment is that the sooner symptoms are identified, the sooner they can be controlled with a few simple precautions.

Taken internally, supplements like vitamin C with bioflavonoids increase capillary strength. B vitamins and especially niacinamide (vitamin B3) keep inflammatory processes under control. Turmeric is another good anti-inflammatory, and astaxantin and lycopene help prevent sun damage that leads to inflammation.

Serums containing vitamin C and niacinamide should be used daily, and when you feel flushed misting with green tea and anti-inflammatories like licorice root will help keep redness at bay.

MOST IMPORTANT OF ALL: DO USE SUNSCREEN

Ideally, you wear sunscreen every day, especially a sunscreen containing zinc oxide. However, many men may be reluctant to wear a sunscreen that shows, and zinc oxide is quite white. Tinted versions can look like makeup, not popular among much of the male population. I sympathize with your dilemma and have been working on formulating a new type of sunscreen that will be virtually invisible.

In the meantime, if you want to reduce redness without applying sunscreen every day, try this out-of-box solution:

USE A SUNSCREEN CONTAINING ZINC OXIDE AT NIGHT. Apply a serum containing vitamin C and niacinamide, then follow with the sunscreen. Zinc combined with niacinamide makes a powerful anti-inflammatory team.

When you wash it off the next morning scrub gently; the remaining zinc oxide will offer protection during the day—and it won't show. After washing, apply a vitamin C and niacinamide serum, and follow with an oil blend that contains astaxanthin, lycopene and other oils from the carotenoid family for a sun protection boost.

RESOURCES:
1. FDA: Topical Acne Products Can Cause Dangerous Side Effects

CLARA:
a SUCCESSFUL
CASE STUDY

WHEN CLARA FIRST CAME TO US

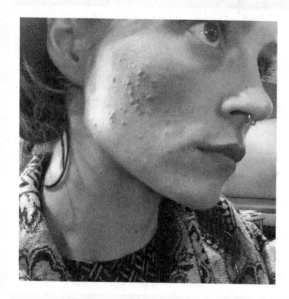

DAY 1:
Extensive, severe
eruptions on cheeks
and forehead

MARIE VERONIQUE Clara had clear, problem-free skin till the age of 32. The onset of acne was very sudden and not accompanied by changes in diet. Clara moved from Seattle to the Bay Area and had stopped an anxiety medication. She consulted a dermatologist, but before trying Accutane or benzoyl peroxide/clindamycin prescriptions she decided to consult us first. Facialist Daniela Sierra directed her treatment path to clear, healthy skin.

CLARA I was trying to minimize my product use completely. I thought everything I used was causing the issues. I changed my diet—cut out meat, dairy, fish, eggs or alcohol. I tried natural/homeopathic remedies, but was afraid to commit to one particular regimen. When I heard about Marie Veronique I was excited to find one product line that was natural and acne-treatment focused. I wanted to start a routine, and when I spoke to Marie personally, she really gave me hope that things were going to be ok.

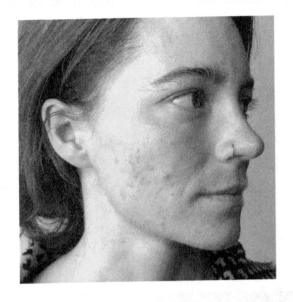

3 MONTHS:
Some improvement
can be seen

SLOW, STEADY PROGRESS

MARIE VERONIQUE After three months of treatment with topicals and some supplementation we can see some improvement, but Clara was feeling frustrated at the slowness of the improvement. We encouraged her to stick with it, knowing this can be the hardest time for people—of course they'd like to see faster results. We also advised increasing the dosage of vitamin B5 and adding n-acetyl carnitine and zinc. Vitamin B5 is water soluble, so you can take quite a lot without risk. (Some of Dr. Leung's patients take up to 20,000 mgs a day.) Adding n-acetyl carnitine, which also helps to break down fats and sebum, significantly decreases the required daily dosage of vitamin B5.

CLARA At first it was a little challenging, the acne came out in full force and it was difficult to look at in the mirror and not pick at my skin. I did, however, understand that things had to get worse before they got better, and Marie and Daniela's positive feedback helped me understand this. The fact is, I saw results rather quickly, rather than the same situation not getting any better; this gave me hope. I was not great about taking the supplements at first, but then later about three months in, I began taking B5 very regularly and that really helped speed up the process, especially with clearing my skin.

SIGNIFICANT IMPROVEMENT

MARIE VERONIQUE After four months of treatment we see significant improvement. Clara is now ready to work on scarring and post-inflammatory hyperpigmentation. We have added a lightening serum to the topical retinol she is using nightly.

CLARA I felt beautiful. For the first time in a year, I was able to look in the mirror and smile rather than frown. I was no longer picking my face apart (literally and figuratively). My confidence and compliments from others came back, which made me feel better and less stressed.

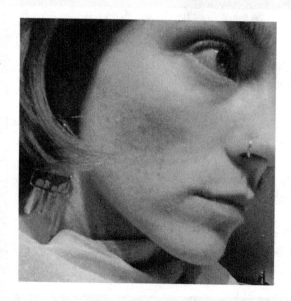

4 MONTHS:
Healing and clearing continues

LASTING RESULTS

MARIE VERONIQUE These last two pictures were taken after six months. They speak for themselves, but I am especially taken by how healthy her skin appears. She says people now ask her what she is doing for her skin because it looks so nice. This is the ultimate compliment, and one I love hearing as much as my clients do.

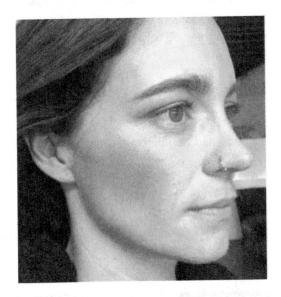

6 MONTHS:
On the road to recovery

SIDE NOTE FROM MARIE

It's been my observation that conventional antibiotic/antimicrobial treatments, while they clear the skin, often leave it dry and dull-looking. And they're not the always the best option for adult acne sufferers who need to consider which treatments may cause premature aging.

CLARA Never in my life would I have known or understood what acne can do to a person's confidence and overall feeling of self.

I feel like my light came back and with even more vibrancy!

I am forever grateful for the treatments that Marie and her team developed, and I have learned so much along the way!

✳ THANK YOU ✳
MARIE and DANIELA

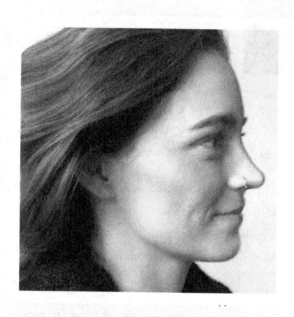

6 MONTHS:
Healthy, glowing
skin following
a natural approach
to acne treatment

EXPERT FACIALIST DANIELA SERRA ON CLARA'S TREATMENT PROTOCOL

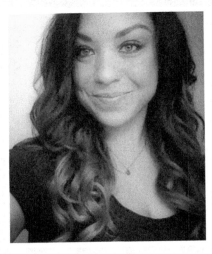

DANIELA SERRA, FACIALIST

We started Clara with facial treatments once a week for four weeks to get her on track. I alternated cleansing mud masks with detoxifying masks and enzymes in order to bring the toxins to the surface of the skin as quickly as possible.

For her home routine, I urged Clara to remain consistent in her use of the treatment cleanser, mist, serum and oil, both morning and night.

AFTER A FEW WEEKS we added retinol serum to aid the repair process. I believe retinol really accelerated the healing and clearing of Clara's skin.

AFTER FOUR CONSECUTIVE WEEKS of facial treatments, I advised Clara that, provided she adhere faithfully to her home routine, we could continue the progress she was making with just one facial a month. We also increased vitamin B5 supplementation at this time, from 500 mgs 2 x a day to 1,000 mgs 3 x a day.

AFTER A FEW MORE MONTHS she was definitely on the road to recovery. The congestion had cleared up, and I was very pleased to see Clara's skin starting to glow. Now all that was left was to repair and heal post-acne scarring and hyperpigmentation.

I added lightening serum to Clara's nightly routine, instructing her to layer lightening serum over the retinol serum every night.

This considerably sped up the healing of residual scarring, as well as evening out the hyperpigmented areas.

CONCLUSION

Routines including supplements and topical products that nourish the skin while protecting healthy microbiota can be used as replacements for, or in addition to, conventional acne treatments.

Natural approaches require a commitment of time and quite a lot of patience on the part of the client, as altering gut and skin microbiomes can take a number of months.

✳ THE UPSIDES ARE WORTH IT ✳

→ ONCE GOOD RESULTS HAVE BEEN ACHIEVED, THEY ARE FAR MORE LIKELY TO BE PERMANENT

→ THE HEALTHY GLOW IS A PLUS. MANY CONVENTIONAL TREATMENTS THAT CLEAR THE SKIN LEAVE IT LOOKING DRY AND DULL. SOMETIMES THERE'S AN ALMOST PLASTIC LOOK TO THE SKIN.

→ NO WORRIES WITH RESPECT TO PREMATURE AGING OR PHOTOSENSITIZATION

→ NO PROBLEMS WITH ANTIBIOTIC RESISTANCE

TREATMENT GUIDELINES

· SECTION ·
TWO

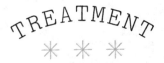

ACNE OVERVIEW

To avoid becoming overwhelmed when you begin your routine, start with simple, beneficial changes. As you see improvement, you'll gain the confidence to add more steps from the Treatment Guidelines to your routine.

The supplements lists are prioritized, with internal changes first, followed by a few topical fixes that will alter the environment of the skin microbiome.

ACNE TIPS

WEAR SUNSCREEN It is seriously important to wear sunscreen daily, and the combination of zinc oxide and niacinamide provides excellent anti-inflammatory action.

If you use a tinted zinc oxide sunscreen you have the best of all worlds—in addition to sun protection you'll have the cosmetic advantage of being able to even out skin tones and conceal redness and inflammation.

ACNE EXTRACTIONS Picking at pimples can drive infection deeper into the hair follicle and infect neighboring follicles by encouraging spread of *Pro-pionibacterium acnes*. You risk permanently compromising the integrity of the follicle walls, so pimples will show up in the same spot over and over again. In extreme cases you can cause scarring.

WHAT TO DO INSTEAD Visit an esthetician skilled at performing extractions without damaging follicles. If you have a lot of comedones, getting them cleared out will hasten the healing process.

Using oil every night keeps pores clear and prevents new pimples from forming.

OLDER ADULTS do not want to use products that generate more free radicals, like benzoyl peroxide. The key is to cure the acne without accelerating aging.

BEST PRACTICES: SUPPLEMENTS

INTERNAL

B VITAMINS Vitamin B deficiency is all too common, and with acne sufferers the need for vitamin B5 is very high.

Everyone can benefit by taking 500 to 1000 mgs of pantothenic acid (vitamin B5) daily. Or try 2 tbsps of nutritional yeast daily, mixed in water or juice.

PROBIOTICS taken internally will help balance gut microbiota. If you're taking antibiotics prescribed by your dermatologist for acne, it's extremely important to add good bacteria into the gut and onto the skin.

FOODS HIGH IN PROBIOTICS are a good place to start, like fermented foods or yogurt, or add powdered probiotics to your juice.

MINERALS and TRACE MINERALS (an ocean source is best) taken internally address deficiencies that might contribute to acne. Most of us are mineral deficient— estimated around 90%.

ABOUT TAKING SUPPLEMENTS The more accustomed you get to taking supplements, see what others you may add according to the treatment guideline that best fits you.

All supplements mentioned are easily found in health food or grocery markets.

TOPICAL

APPLE CIDER VINEGAR keeps friendly microbes happy by helping skin maintain a low pH. A splash in your rinse water after you cleanse at night will lower your pH to levels that commensal microbes like and that pathogens like *Staphylococcus aureus* do not.

FULL-FAT PLAIN YOGURT is a great multitasker. Check the yogurt label to make sure it contains live bacterial cultures.

TO CLEANSE Take ¼ tsp of yogurt, spread over face, rinse. To use as a mask: Simply leave on your ¼ tsp yogurt for 10-15 minutes before rinsing.

→ AVOID ANTI-ACNE CLEANSERS CONTAINING TRICLOSAN OR BENZOYL PEROXIDE. THEY CAUSE MICROBIAL DISRUPTION—WHAT YOU WANT IS MICROBIAL BALANCE

TO MOISTURIZE Spread a thin layer, about ⅛ tsp, over entire face and leave on overnight.

→ AVOID MOISTURIZERS CONTAINING WAX AND/OR TOO MANY ANTIMICROBIALS, AND OIL-FREE MOISTURIZERS

SUNFLOWER AND SAFFLOWER OILS make excellent exfoliators that do not strip skin. Oils have the ability to clear congestion because they penetrate more deeply and dissolve compacted matter (oils dissolve oils).

Once or twice a week, massage a dime-sized drop of oil directly into your skin. No need to rinse. Oils high in omega-6 essential fatty acids like safflower and sunflower are the best, especially for the folks who produce a type of sticky sebum, low in omega-6 EFAs, that clogs pores.

ROSACEA IS NOT ACNE

Rosacea originates from defective innate immune system responses. However, it can resemble acne and has been called "acne rosacea." Treating it with anti-acne medications can increase inflammation and worsen the condition.

Because rosacea has symptoms in common with a number of serious diseases like lupus, it must be diagnosed by a qualified health professional prior to beginning treatment.

|| FOR ROSACEA-SPECIFIC TREATMENT DETAILS, SEE ||
|| PAGES 126-139

ADULT ACNE: WOMEN

FOR WOMEN WITH MILD TO MODERATE ACNE, characterized by blackheads, whiteheads and occasional breakouts.

✳ WEEKLY ROUTINE ✳

Use exfoliating mask once or twice a week, at night only, but be careful not to over-dry the skin. Look for a mask with lactic acid, salicylic acid, malic acid, and enzymes in papaya, pineapple and pumpkin. Follow with an oil blend.

✳ SUNSCREEN NOTE ✳

Everyone should wear sunscreen daily, particularly one with zinc oxide. If you are reluctant to wear a sunscreen that shows, and zinc oxide is quite white, an alternative is to wear it at night instead. Zinc, combined with niacinamide makes a powerful anti-inflammatory team.

Wash off gently the next morning—remaining zinc oxide will continue to protect during the day, invisibly!

MORNING ROUTINE

№ 1 CLEANSE WITH A MILD GEL OR OIL-BASED
Avoid soaps; they are too drying and alkaline

№ 2 HYDRATE WITH A LOW pH MIST containing
anti-inflammatories like licorice root or green tea

№ 3 APPLY A SERUM RICH IN VITAMINS C AND E

№ 4 MASSAGE IN AN OIL HIGH IN OMEGA 6s AND 3s

№ 5 APPLY ZINC OXIDE SUNSCREEN

NIGHT ROUTINE

№ 1 CLEANSE WITH A MILD GEL OR OIL-BASED CLEANSER
Avoid soaps; they are too drying and alkaline

№ 2 HYDRATE WITH A LOW pH MIST containing
anti-inflammatories like licorice root or green tea

№ 3 MASSAGE IN AN OIL HIGH IN OMEGA 6s AND 3s
while face is still damp

№ 4 APPLY A NIANCINAMIDE/PANTOTHENIC ACID SERUM

№ 5 APPLY A RETINOL SERUM

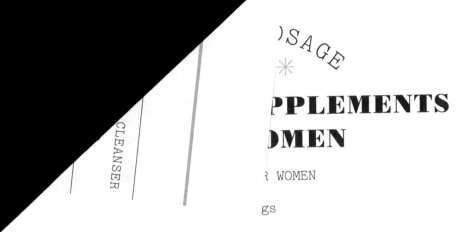

→ VITAMIN Bs / 1-2 B-Complex capsules
or ANY NUTRITIONAL YEAST / 1-2 tbsps

→ VITAMIN B5 / 1,000-2,000mgs in AM/PM 500mg doses
Vitamin B5 is water soluble, so you can't take too much.

→ ACETYL L-CARNITINE / 500mgs
To help with sebum breakdown.

→ NIACINAMIDE or VITAMIN B3 / 500mgs

→ OMEGA 3: FISH or KRILL OIL / 1-2 tbsps
or KRILL CAPSULES / 1-2

→ PROBIOTICS
Take a probiotic supplement to improve digestion. Supplementing good
bacteria in the gut with probiotics will optimize value of the supplement
regime, since microbes are instrumental in making vitamins.

TREATMENT TRUTHS: DOWNSIDES of DEEP CLEANSING

You've tried everything, but your acne gets worse. Your skin is drier than ever and new wrinkles start to surface. Sound familiar?

From teen years on, we were told that oil- and dirt-clogged pores cause acne and that the best treatments are "deep cleansing" and daily exfoliation. We now know that cleansing with harsh surfactants, excessive peels and scraping away rather than replenishing the precious stratum corneum contribute to the dryness and aggravate breakouts—especially with adults. We also know that oils help keep skin both youthful and blemish-free.

3 WAYS TO RETHINK YOUR ROUTINE

STOP excessive deep-cleansing activities, like peels more than once a week. Avoid sonic cleansers and gadgets altogether.

WHY Oils protect against bacterial attack—and keep skin soft and supple.

STOP insisting on all oil-free products.

WHY Oils penetrate well and reach the source of the congestion.

STOP using conventional exfoliants that only scratch the surface, literally.

WHY Because oil dissolves oil, oil exfoliants break up congestion where it starts, deep in the pores, and return EFAs to the skin.

ADULT ACNE: MEN

FOR MEN WITH OILY SKIN AND/OR MILD TO MODERATE ACNE. characterized by blackheads, whiteheads and occasional breakouts. Thanks to testosterone, men's skin differs from women's skin. Because men have a higher concentration of blood vessels, excessive sebum production, thicker skin and more facial hair, the following treatments were developed to target men's unique skin conditions: razor bumps, blemishes and breakouts into adulthood, and excessive redness.

✳ SUNSCREEN NOTE ✳

Everyone should wear sunscreen daily, particularly one with zinc oxide. If you are reluctant to wear a sunscreen that shows, and zinc oxide is quite white, an alternative is to wear it at night instead. Zinc, combined with niacinamide makes a powerful anti-inflammatory team.

Wash off gently the next morning—remaining zinc oxide will continue to protect during the day, invisibly!

MORNING ROUTINE

№ 1 CLEANSE WITH A MILD GEL OR SOAP

№ 2 HYDRATE WITH A LOW pH MIST containing
anti-inflammatories like licorice root or green tea,
or splash on lightly diluted apple cider vinegar

№ 3 APPLY A SERUM RICH IN VITAMINS C AND E

№ 4 MASSAGE IN AN OIL HIGH IN OMEGA 6s AND 3s

№ 5 BEST PRACTICE: APPLY ZINC OXIDE SUNSCREEN

NIGHT ROUTINE

№ 1 CLEANSE WITH A MILD GEL OR OIL-BASED CLEANSER
You may use a cleanser containing salicylic acid

№ 2 HYDRATE WITH A LOW pH MIST containing
anti-inflammatories like licorice root or green tea,
or splash on lightly diluted apple cider vinegar

№ 3 MASSAGE IN AN OIL HIGH IN OMEGA 6s AND 3s
while face is still damp

№ 4 APPLY A RETINOL SERUM OR RETINOID PRODUCT
prescribed by a dermatologist

№ 5 APPLY A RETINOL SERUM

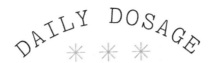

INTERNAL SUPPLEMENTS FOR MEN

→ MULTIVITAMIN DESIGNED FOR MEN

→ VITAMIN C / 1,000-2,000mgs

→ VITAMIN E / 400IUS

→ VITAMIN Bs / 1-2 B-Complex capsules
or ANY NUTRITIONAL YEAST / 1-2 tbsps

→ VITAMIN B5 / 2,000-4,000mgs in AM/PM 500mg doses
Vitamin B5 is water soluble, so you can't take too much.

→ ACETYL L-CARNITINE / 1000mgs
To help with sebum breakdown.

→ NIACINAMIDE or VITAMIN B3 / 500mgs

→ OMEGA 3: FISH or KRILL OIL / 1-2 tbsps
or KRILL CAPSULES / 1-2

→ PROBIOTICS
Take a probiotic supplement to improve digestion. Supplementing good
bacteria in the gut with probiotics will optimize value of the supplement
regime, since microbes are instrumental in making vitamins.

SHAVING BEST PRACTICES

→ EXFOLIATE THE SKIN
with a cleanser containing salicylic acid.

→ USE WARM WATER TO RINSE OFF THE CLEANSER
Keep your face moistened to soften coarse hair.

→ LATHER UP WITH A MOISTURIZING SHAVING CREAM OR GEL

→ ALWAYS SHAVE IN THE DIRECTION THE HAIR GROWS
Use as few strokes possible; avoid stretching skin.

→ SPLASH ON A BIT OF APPLE CIDER VINEGAR AFTER SHAVING
Do not use alcohol, which dries the skin.

→ FOLLOW WITH AN OIL BLEND TO PREVENT CLOGGED PORES
*Do not use an oil-free moisturizer; oils are essential
to keep pores clear.*

ACNE VULGARIS: ADOLESCENTS & ADULTS, MEN & WOMEN

SEVERE ACNE NEEDS TO BE TREATED UNDER THE SKILLED SUPERVISION OF A DERMATOLOGIST. These recommendations can be integrated into the anti-acne program recommended by your doctor.

✳ SUNSCREEN NOTE ✳

It is seriously important to wear sunscreen daily, and the combination of zinc oxide and niacinamide provides excellent anti-inflammatory action. If you use a tinted zinc oxide sunscreen you have the best of all worlds—in addition to sun protection you'll have the cosmetic advantage of being able to even out skin tones and conceal redness and inflammation.

MORNING ROUTINE

№ 1 CLEANSE WITH A MILD GEL OR SOAP
Preferably a soap containing salicylic acid, if
you're not allergic. If you are, use a cleanser
containing lactic acid or malic acid. Avoid glycolic
acid because it can trigger hyperpigmentation.

№ 2 HYDRATE WITH A LOW pH MIST containing
anti-inflammatories like licorice root or green tea,
or splash on a little apple cider vinegar. You may
want to dilute the vinegar's strength with water.

№ 3 APPLY A SERUM RICH IN VITAMINS C AND E
You may also use a spot treatment serum for particularly troublesome areas.

№ 4 MASSAGE IN AN OIL HIGH IN OMEGA 6s AND 3s

№ 5 APPLY ZINC OXIDE SUNSCREEN

NIGHT ROUTINE

№ 1 CLEANSE WITH A MILD GEL OR OIL-BASED CLEANSER
You may use a cleanser containing salicylic acid.

№ 2 HYDRATE WITH A LOW pH MIST containing
anti-inflammatories like licorice root or green tea,
or splash on water-diluted apple cider vinegar.

№ 3 APPLY A VITAMINS B3/B5 SERUM

№ 4 APPLY A RETINOL SERUM OR RETINOID PRODUCT
prescribed by a dermatologist.

№ 5 MASSAGE IN AN OIL HIGH IN OMEGA 6s AND 3s

SHAVING BEST PRACTICES

→ EXFOLIATE THE SKIN
with a cleanser containing salicylic acid.

→ USE WARM WATER TO RINSE OFF THE CLEANSER
Keep your face moistened to soften coarse hair.

→ LATHER UP WITH A MOISTURIZING SHAVING CREAM OR GEL

→ ALWAYS SHAVE IN THE DIRECTION THE HAIR GROWS
Use as few strokes possible; avoid stretching skin.

→ SPLASH ON A BIT OF APPLE CIDER VINEGAR AFTER SHAVING
Do not use alcohol, which dries the skin.

→ FOLLOW WITH AN OIL BLEND TO PREVENT CLOGGED PORES
*Do not use an oil-free moisturizer; oils are essential
to keep pores clear.*

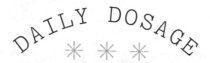

INTERNAL SUPPLEMENTS FOR ACNE VULGARIS

→ ONE MULTIVITAMIN

→ VITAMIN C / 1,000-2,000mgs

→ VITAMIN E / 400IUS

→ VITAMIN Bs / 1-2 B-Complex capsules
or ANY NUTRITIONAL YEAST / 1-2 tbsps

→ VITAMIN B5 / 4,000-8,000mgs in AM/PM 500mg doses
Vitamin B5 is water soluble, so you can't take too much.

→ ACETYL L-CARNITINE / 1000mgs
To help with sebum breakdown.

→ NIACINAMIDE or VITAMIN B3 / 500mgs

→ OMEGA 3: FISH or KRILL OIL / 1-2 tbsps
or KRILL CAPSULES / 1-2

→ MINERALS AND TRACE MINERALS (ocean source is best)
Helps take care of deficiencies that might contribute to acne. Most of us are mineral deficient—estimated around 90%.

→ PROBIOTICS / food-based or 1-2/day with meals
Taking probiotics internally will help balance gut microbiota. If taking antibiotics prescribed by your dermatologist for your acne it is extremely important that you make sure you add "good" bacteria into the gut and onto the skin. Probiotics are found in foods like fermented vegetables and yogurt. You may also take capsules, 1-2 a day, with meals.

✳ WOMEN WITH PCOS ✳
POLYCYCSTIC OVARIAN SYNDROME

Women who have PCOS, approximately 6-10% of all women, typically have high levels of androgens—male hormones normally produced in small amounts in all women's bodies.

The cause is unknown. Here is some additional supplemental advice for women struggling with PCOS.

FLAXSEED contains lignans that increase the production of sex hormone-binding globulin (SHBG) that binds testosterone in the blood.

→ Daily: Mix 1 or 2 tbsps of freshly ground flaxseeds in a glass of water.

SPEARMINT TEA reduces testosterone levels by increasing luteinizing hormone (LH) and follicle-stimulating hormone (FSH) levels.

→ Add 1 tsp dried spearmint leaves to 1 cup boiled water and let steep for 5-10 minutes. Drink 1-2 cups daily.

SAW PALMETTO This herb acts as an anti-androgen, blocks 5-alpha-reductase activity and reduces the conversion of testosterone into a more active form called dihydrotestosterone (DHT).

→ Take 320 mg of standardized saw palmetto extract daily for a few months. If you are taking a liquid extract, take 1 tsp per day.

OMEGA-3 Some research indicates supplementing omega 3s and 6s can decrease androgen levels in women with PCOS.

One study found that women with PCOS who were given three grams of omega 3s a day for eight weeks had lower testosterone concentrations and were more likely to resume regular menses than subjects who received a placebo.

→ Increase fish oil intake to 3 tbsps a day.

INOSITOL supplementation is sometimes used to regulate endocrine disorders, specifically PCOS. Two inositol isomers, myo-inositol (MI) and D-Chiro-inositol (DCI) have proven to be effective in PCOS treatment by improving insulin resistance, serum androgen levels and many features of the metabolic syndrome.

PCOS women appeared to get some benefit from a dose of only 200 mg daily, which is a very moderate amount. Some doctors may recommend 500 mg twice daily. In contrast, as much as 12 grams (12,000 mg) has been used in studies to treat depression or panic attacks.

→ 200-1,000 mg per day for PCOS appears safe, as it is water soluble. Regular inositol is inexpensive and available in capsules, tablets or powder.

D-CHIRO-INOSITOL (DCI) is a member of a family of related substances often referred to collectively as "inositol." Though not abundant in most diets, it is found in small quantities in buckwheat.

→ Add buckwheat to your diet and take a suitable inositol (MI) supplement, in place of expensive supplements with a ratio of 2000 MI to 40 DI.

APPROACH WITH CAUTION

BENZOYL PEROXIDE generates free radicals and accelerates aging, but for teens with acne BP can be effective, as it is quite successful in killing *P. acnes*. If you do decide to use BP, proceed cautiously and follow these tips.

If you don't respond quickly, discontinue use. BP is not for everyone.

If you can use it successfully, once your skin is clear ease off the use by introducing oil blends, tea tree oil and B5 serums instead.

It's good to begin easing off early in the game, because there usually comes a time when BP stops working. People are advised to curtail use for a while, but then the acne tends to come back with a vengeance. Sometimes people are advised to use higher concentrations to avoid the return of the acne, but this follows the law of diminishing returns—and you end up stuck in a vicious cycle of needing more to get fewer positive results.

Be aware that there is an end game to BP use, and it's best not to become too dependent on it.

BP IS A PHOTOSENSITIZER ✳ ALWAYS WEAR SUNSCREEN ✳ WHEN USING BP PRODUCTS

The FDA has issued a warning against benzoyl peroxide, which can cause severe allergic reactions in some people.

IF YOU EXPERIENCE ANY of THESE SYMPTOMS, DISCONTINUE BP USE IMMEDIATELY

→ THROAT TIGHTNESS

→ SHORTNESS OF BREATH, WHEEZING

→ LOW BLOOD PRESSURE

→ FAINTING OR COLLAPSE

→ HIVES

→ ITCHING OF FACE OR BODY

→ SWELLING OF EYES, FACE, LIPS

AVOID COMPLETELY

ANTI-ACNE CLEANSERS CONTAINING TRICLOSAN In addition to studies that link triclosan to a range of health and environmental effects, from skin irritation, allergy susceptibility and bacterial resistance to dioxin contamination of fragile aquatic ecosystems, other studies show that it isn't any more effective in combating germs than plain soap and water. Too much triclosan can disrupt microbial balance and by killing off too many "helper" bacteria make skin vulnerable to pathogenic invasion. Ultimately, triclosan overuse could lead to trading a case of pimples for an eruption of boils.

ANTI-ACNE CLEANSERS CONTAINING ALCOHOL Alcohol irritates and dries skin, and increases sebum production. It is also a microbial disruptor, creating conditions of irritation and microbial imbalance, which could invite pathogenic assault.

TREATMENT

✳ ✳ ✳

ROSACEA OVERVIEW

‖ ROSACEA MUST BE PROPERLY DIAGNOSED BEFORE ‖
‖ PROCEEDING WITH TREATMENT ‖

Many serious diseases such as lupus have symptoms in common with rosacea, and a qualified health professional is required to make an accurate diagnosis. Know what you're dealing with before you embark on any treatment.

ROSACEA AND ACNE

Later stages of rosacea may prompt rashes or eruptions that look like pimples. However, they are not pimples and should never be treated as such.

PERFORMING EXTRACTIONS will increase inflammation. Try anti-inflammatory techniques instead.

TOPICAL MEDICATIONS

ANTIBIOTICS Rosacea sufferers are often prescribed antibiotic creams such as metronidazole and clindamycin. Even though bacteria is not the cause, the abnormal cathelicidin peptides that initiate the symptoms of rosacea are alleviated by antibiotics that seem to inhibit the enzymes.

IMMUNE RESPONSE Since bacteria aren't the targets, treatments that modulate the immune response make more sense. To that end, avoid triggers that set off the immune response, most notably:

IMMUNE RESPONSE TRIGGERS

→ UV EXPOSURE AND/OR HEAT

→ ANTIMICROBIAL SOAPS AND TOPICAL TREATMENTS
 that may disrupt microbial balance

→ TONERS CONTAINING ALCOHOL OR ASTRINGENTS

→ CHEMICAL SUNSCREENS

→ BENZOYL PEROXIDE

WHAT ABOUT ALCOHOL, CAFFEINE and SPICY FOODS?

W. C. Fields' red nose was an advanced case of rhinophyma, but since he was also an alcoholic, the common misconception was to blame drinking for his condition.

Little wonder, many people are surprised to learn that rosacea is not caused by alcoholism at all. Imbibing alcohol can exacerbate an existing rosacea condition, but lifelong teetotalers can suffer equally severe rosacea.

So, what to do if alcohol appears to be one your triggers? Or caffeine or spicy foods for that matter, which many of us consider the finer things in life?

Common sense says moderation can promote a longer, healthier life. However, abjuring things you enjoy may not necessarily help clear your rosacea. On the other hand, occasional food and drink indulgences can relieve stress, a known and very significant rosacea trigger.

TREATMENT for MITES

Rosacea sufferers tend to be generous hosts to *Human Demodex*, the mite that lives in hair follicles. The population is about 50% denser in rosacea-prone people, and recent studies indicate that the link between mite populations and rosacea is quite real.

It may not necessarily be the causative factor, but if you feel that mites just might be a problem, try these recipes.

MITICIDE FACIAL SCRUB/MASK

→ GREEN MUNG BEANS, coarsely ground, 50 g

→ NEEM LEAF, finely sieved powder, 50 g

→ WHITE SANDALWOOD, finely sieved powder, 50 g

→ NEEM OIL, 25 ml

GENTLE SCRUB Mix all ingredients together, and use a small handful with a little bit of water to make a paste. Use the paste as a facial scrub, gently rubbing the mixture over the affected area to exfoliate and remove the mites.

USE THIS SCRUB TO CONTROL BLEPHARITIS in the same way, but apply very gently between the lashes with a cotton swab, then rinse.

MASK If the area is too sensitive or irritated to use as a scrub, apply the paste over the affected areas. Leave on for 15-20 minutes, then remove with water.

Gentle enough to use daily, in the evening.

TEA TREE OIL

Tea tree oil is an excellent miticide. Use tea tree soap or face wash daily.

In addition to commercial products, you can make an oil blend with up to 25% tea tree oil to apply to the skin.

The concentration of tea tree oil purportedly needs to be 50% to be effective, however this is very strong and will burn the skin. I recommend using a 25% solution of tea tree oil and adding 25% neem oil, another effective miticide that is less irritating.

If you have blepharitis and use this blend to kill eyelash mites, apply a tiny amount on a cotton swab, careful not to let it get into your eyes—it will sting.

MITICIDE OIL RECIPE

→   JOJOBA, SAFFLOWER OR SUNFLOWER OIL, 25 ml

→   TEA TREE OIL, 25 ml

→   SEA BUCKTHORN OIL, 25 ml

→   NEEM OIL, 25 ml

Mix ingredients together. Store in a cool place. Shake well before using.

Mites come out at night to mate when it's dark, so the best time to apply a tiny amount to the affected areas is just before bedtime.

If you do have an infestation, you may feel some perturbation from the critters encountering and reacting to the oil.

PROBIOTICS The rosacea-type immune system response to invading microorganisms creates inflammation resulting in redness and bumps. Topically applied probiotics can help provide bacterial interference, antimicrobial peptides and a calming effect.

YOGURT, OATMEAL & TURMERIC CLEANSER/MASK

→ WHOLE MILK YOGURT, 1-2 cups

→ GROUND OATMEAL, ¼ cup

→ TURMERIC, ½ tsp

Grind oatmeal in a blender to make a fine powder. Mix with yogurt and turmeric to make a paste. Store in a covered glass container. Keep refrigerated.

As a cleanser, take ½ tsp of the paste and gently apply all over face; rinse with warm water. To use as a mask, apply the same amount and leave on for 10-15 minutes; rinse with warm water.

Plain yogurt can also be used as a moisturizer. Apply a very thin layer, just enough so it disappears into the skin, about ⅛ tsp. Let dry. Cover with sunscreen in the morning, and at night follow the yogurt layer with serums as usual.

GREEN TEA MIST

Steep 4-5 green tea bags in 1 qt water. Let cool. Pour into a mist bottle and spray it on morning and night as part of your routine. Mist any time your skin needs calming. It's indispensable whenever you're outdoors.

✳ FUN FACTS about MITES ✳

№ 1 Mites are relatives of ticks, spiders, scorpions and other arachnids. Over 48,000 species have been described, but many millions more are yet to be identified. They are highly specialized, many are parasites, and they're particular about their hosts.

№ 2 One mite lives only on the eyeballs of a certain fruit bat, there's another that chooses to live only in the anus of a sloth, and then there are two out of the 65 belonging to the genus *Demodex*; *D. folliculorum* and *D. brevis*, who have chosen to live on humans and humans alone.

№ 3 *Demodex folliculorum* are the fun-loving mites. They crawl out of their sebaceous glands at night to mate, then return to their pores when dawn breaks or when they've had enough.

They like to lay their eggs on the rims of your eyelashes (something to think about the next time you sleepily rub your eyes at night.)

№ 4 *D. folliculorum* have developed a unique way of going out with a bang as well. Lacking an anus they just store all their waste matter up until the moment of death, at which point they explode it all over your face.

№ 5 This rather nasty habit of theirs just might be the connection between rosacea and *Demodex*, because if you are harboring a good many mites, excessive amounts of waste products on your skin might trigger an immune system response setting off an inflammatory cascade.

ROSACEA: WOMEN

ROSACEA MUST BE DIAGNOSED BEFORE PROCEEDING WITH TREATMENT. Many serious diseases such as lupus have symptoms in common with rosacea, and a qualified health professional is required to make an accurate diagnosis. Know what you're dealing with before you embark on any treatment.

MORNING ROUTINE

№ 1 CLEANSE WITH TEPID WATER OR YOGURT
Avoid soaps; they are too drying and alkaline

№ 2 HYDRATE WITH A LOW pH MIST containing
anti-inflammatories like licorice root or green tea

№ 3 APPLY A VITAMINS C, E AND NIACINAMIDE SERUM

№ 4 MASSAGE IN AN OIL HIGH IN OMEGA 6s AND 3s

№ 5 APPLY ZINC OXIDE SUNSCREEN

NIGHT ROUTINE

№ 1 CLEANSE WITH YOGURT, A MILD GEL OR OIL-BASED CLEANSER Avoid soaps; they are too drying and alkaline

№ 2 HYDRATE WITH A LOW pH MIST containing anti-inflammatories like licorice root or green tea

№ 3 YOU MAY USE YOGURT AS A MOISTURIZER Apply about ¼ tsp all over face, let dry, then layer a serum containing niacinamide

№ 4 APPLY A RETINOL SERUM

№ 5 MASSAGE IN AN OIL HIGH IN OMEGA 6s AND 3s

✳ ROSACEA MASK FOR WOMEN ✳

You may use a yogurt mask every night. Simply apply about ½ tsp yogurt to face and neck, let dry—about 10-15 minutes, then rinse with tepid water. That's it!

A MORE ELABORATE YOGURT MASK To 2-3 tbsp yogurt: Add ½ tsp ground oatmeal, ½ tsp ground flaxseed and a dash of turmeric. Apply ¼-½ tsp all over face and neck, let dry about 10-15 minutes, then rinse. Store the rest in the refrigerator. May be used nightly. Continue with your regular nighttime routine after use.

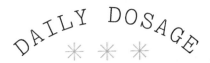

INTERNAL SUPPLEMENTS
WOMEN WITH ROSACEA

→ MULTIVITAMIN DESIGNED FOR WOMEN

→ VITAMIN C WITH BIOFLAVONOIDS / 500mgs, 2 x day

→ VITAMIN E / 400IUS

→ NIACINAMIDE / 500mgs

→ ANTIOXIDANTS ASTAXANTHIN &/OR LYCOPENE / 1 capsule

→ CURCUMIN / 500mgs

→ OMEGA-3 EFAS: FISH or KRILL OIL / 1-2 tbsps
or KRILL CAPSULES / 1-2
Eicosapentaenoic acid (EPA) can be found in some algae oils as well.

→ GREEN TEA EXTRACT
Look for compound epigallocatechin gallate (ECGC).

→ VITAMIN B5 / 1,000-2,000mgs in AM/PM 500mg doses
Vitamin B5 is water soluble, so you can't take too much.

→ PROBIOTICS
Supplement good bacteria in the gut with probiotics to improve digestion and optimize value; microbes are essential in making vitamins.

→ MINERALS AND TRACE MINERALS
Deficiencies contribute to inflammation. The sea is the best source for all minerals needed; balanced proportions are predetermined by nature.

TREATMENT GUIDELINES

NIACINAMIDE & ZINC

Both of these powerful anti-inflammatories are being studied for their efficacy in treating inflammatory diseases like rosacea and acne vulgaris. Combined as a lotion, niacinamide (derived from vitamin B3) and zinc oxide make not only an effective moisturizer and skin shield, but also help relieve swelling and inflammation.

NIACINAMIDE AND ZINC LOTION

At night, combine a pea-sized amount of serum containing niacinamde with a similar amount of your zinc oxide sunscreen in the palm of your hand. Apply as the final step of your nightly routine.

ROSACEA: MEN

ROSACEA MUST BE DIAGNOSED before proceeding with treatment. Serious diseases such as lupus have symptoms in common with rosacea, and a qualified health professional is required to make an accurate diagnosis.

Because of the higher concentration of blood vessels, particularly on the cheekbones, many men appear to have permanently red faces. After all, redness may be the first sign of developing rosacea, and the cause of all types of redness is hyper-reactivity of the skin's vessels.

ROSACEA AFFECTS MEN AND WOMEN SOMEWHAT DIFFERENTLY. Redness, proliferation of the sebaceous glands and swelling of the skin on the nose (rhinophyma, a condition found in advanced rosacea) is nearly exclusive to males.

I encourage you to consult a physician well before a serious condition like rhinophyma develops. The preponderance of advanced cases of rosacea among men can be attributed to not proactively catching it at an early stage. When it comes to rosacea an ounce of prevention is worth a pound of cure—and for rhino-phyma there is no cure! If you have rosacea follow the daily routines and add the suggested masks and supplementation as well.

✳ SUNSCREEN NOTE ✳

Everyone should wear sunscreen daily, particularly one with zinc oxide. If you are reluctant to wear a sunscreen that shows, and zinc oxide is quite white, an alternative is to wear it at night instead. Zinc, combined with niacinamide makes a powerful anti-inflammatory team.

Wash off gently the next morning—remaining zinc oxide will continue to pro-tect during the day, invisibly!

MORNING ROUTINE

№ 1 CLEANSE WITH TEPID WATER OR YOGURT
Avoid soaps; they are too drying and alkaline

№ 2 HYDRATE WITH A LOW pH MIST containing anti-inflammatories like licorice root or green tea

№ 3 APPLY A VITAMINS C, E AND NIACINAMIDE SERUM

№ 4 MASSAGE IN AN OIL HIGH IN OMEGA 6s AND 3s

№ 5 APPLY ZINC OXIDE SUNSCREEN

NIGHT ROUTINE

№ 1 CLEANSE WITH YOGURT, A MILD GEL OR OIL-BASED CLEANSER Avoid soaps; they are too drying and alkaline

№ 2 HYDRATE WITH A LOW pH MIST containing anti-inflammatories like licorice root or green tea

№ 3 USE YOGURT AS A MOISTURIZER
Apply about ¼ tsp all over face, let dry, then apply a serum with niacinamide

№ 4 APPLY A RETINOL SERUM or a RETINOID PRODUCT prescribed by your dermatologist

№ 5 MASSAGE IN AN OIL HIGH IN OMEGA 6s AND 3s

№ 6 APPLY ZINC OXIDE SUNSCREEN (OPTIONAL, SEE BELOW)

ROSACEA MASk FOR MEN

You may use a yogurt mask every night. Simply apply about ½ tsp yogurt to face and neck, let dry—about 10-15 minutes, then rinse with tepid water.

A MORE ELABORATE YOGURT MASK To 2-3 tbsp yogurt: Add ½ tsp ground oatmeal, ½ tsp ground flaxseed and a dash of turmeric. Apply ¼-½ tsp all over face and neck, let dry about 10-15 minutes, then rinse. Store the rest in the refrigerator. May be used nightly. Continue with your regular nighttime routine after use.

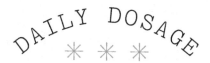

DAILY DOSAGE
* * *

INTERNAL SUPPLEMENTS MEN WITH ROSACEA

→ MULTIVITAMIN DESIGNED FOR MEN

→ VITAMIN C WITH BIOFLAVONOIDS / 500mgs, 2 x day

→ VITAMIN E / 400IUS

→ NIACINAMIDE / 500-1,000mgs, 1-2 x day

→ PANTOTHENIC ACID / 500-1,000mgs

→ ANTIOXIDANTS ASTAXANTHIN &/OR LYCOPENE / 1 capsule

→ CURCUMIN / 500mgs

→ OMEGA-3 EFAS: FISH or KRILL OIL / 1-2 tbsps
or KRILL / 1-2 capsules
Eicosapentaenoic acid (EPA) can be found in some algae oils as well.

→ GREEN TEA EXTRACT
Look for compound epigallocatechin gallate (ECGC).

→ PROBIOTICS
Supplement good bacteria in the gut with probiotics to improve digestion and optimize value; microbes are essential in making vitamins.

→ MINERALS AND TRACE MINERALS
Deficiencies contribute to inflammation. The sea is the best source for
needed minerals; balanced proportions are predetermined by nature.

HYPERPIGMENTATION

LIKE ACNE AND ROSACEA, HYPERPIGMENTATION HAS ITS ORIGIN IN INFLAMMATION. Cases of hyperpigmentation have been increasing in younger and younger people, and we can begin to pinpoint culprits like overuse of antimicrobials and climate change as probable causes.

№ 1 CAUSE OF HYPERPIGMENTATION, SUN DAMAGE from UVA rays—can be prevented with zinc oxide sunscreen. Avoid chemical sunscreens, especially if they contain oxybenzone, octinoxate, octocrylene and avobenzone that break down in the presence of UV to produce free radicals.

ENVIRONMENTAL TRIGGERS

Environmental factors that can trigger inflammation and hyperpigmentation:

→ **SOOT** If you live in a highly polluted area, wash off the soot ASAP

→ **UVA RAYS** penetrate to the dermis, damage DNA and cause hyperpigmentation and broken capillaries

→ **HEAT** Thermal heat signals the skin to produce more melanin

→ **ENVIRONMENTAL POLLUTION**[1] Increase in soot
was associated with 20% more pigment spots on forehead and cheeks

MORNING ROUTINE

№ 1 CLEANSE WITH TEPID WATER OR YOGURT
Avoid soaps; they are too drying and alkaline

№ 2 HYDRATE WITH A LOW pH MIST containing
anti-inflammatories like licorice root or green tea

№ 3 APPLY A VITAMINS C, E AND NIACINAMIDE SERUM

№ 4 MASSAGE IN AN OIL HIGH IN OMEGA 6s AND 3s

№ 5 APPLY ZINC OXIDE SUNSCREEN
Apply liberally if you live in a high-pollution area to
protect against soot penetrating to the stratum corneum

NIGHT ROUTINE

№ 1 CLEANSE WITH YOGURT, MILD GEL OR OIL-BASED CLEANSER
If you live in a highly polluted area, wash off the
soot ASAP to prevent hyperpigmentation from developing.
Avoid soaps; they are too drying and alkaline.

№ 2 HYDRATE WITH A LOW pH MIST containing anti-inflammatories like licorice root or green tea

№ 3 USE YOGURT AS A MOISTURIZER
Apply about ¼ tsp all over face, let dry, then apply a serum with niacinamide and vitamin C

№ 4 APPLY A RETINOL SERUM or a RETINOID PRODUCT prescribed by your dermatologist

---

№ 5 MASSAGE IN AN OIL HIGH IN OMEGA 6s AND 3s

~~~~~~

✳ HYPERPIGMENTATION MASK ✳

You may use a yogurt mask every night. Simply apply about ½ tsp yogurt to face and neck, let dry—about 10-15 minutes, then rinse with tepid water.

A MORE ELABORATE YOGURT MASK To 2-3 tbsp yogurt: Add ½ tsp ground oatmeal, ½ tsp ground flaxseed and a dash of turmeric. Apply ¼-½ tsp all over face and neck, let dry about 10-15 minutes, then rinse.

Store the rest in the refrigerator. May be used nightly. Continue with your regular nighttime routine after use.

LEMON JUICE SCRUB

Cut a fresh lemon into quarters. Rub one of the quarters all over skin for 30 seconds, then rinse off with tepid water. Repeat 2-3x a week.

~~~~~~

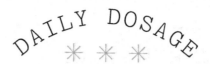

INTERNAL SUPPLEMENTS
HYPERPIGMENTATION

→ MULTIVITAMIN

→ VITAMIN C WITH BIOFLAVONOIDS / 500mgs, 2 x day

→ VITAMIN E / 400IUS

→ NIACINAMIDE / 500mgs

→ ANTIOXIDANTS ASTAXANTHIN &/OR LYCOPENE / 1 capsule

→ CURCUMIN / 500mgs

→ OMEGA-3 EFAS: FISH or KRILL OIL / 1-2 tbsps
or KRILL CAPSULES / 1-2
Eicosapentaenoic acid (EPA) can be found in some algae oils as well.

→ GREEN TEA EXTRACT
Look for compound epigallocatechin gallate (ECGC).

→ PROBIOTICS
Supplement good bacteria in the gut with probiotics to improve digestion and optimize value; microbes are essential in making vitamins.

→ MINERALS AND TRACE MINERALS
Deficiencies contribute to inflammation. The sea is the best source for all minerals that are needed; balanced proportions are predetermined by nature.

HYPERPIGMENTATION VARIETIES

POST-INFLAMMATORY HYPERPIGMENTATION (PIH) Picking at a pimple can eventually lead to scarring and hyperpigmentation.

Acne is the most common cause of PIH, though other causes include psoriasis or a burn. PIH and acne can be treated simultaneously with topical retinoids.

MELASMA Sometimes called "the pregnancy mask" because it occurs routinely in pregnant women, melasma appears as brown to dark brown patches on the face.

It is hormonal–related and usually, but not always, disappears post-partum. Like PIH it affects deeper layers of the skin and thus is harder to treat. Topical retinoids are probably your best bet.

✳ AVOID COMPLETELY ✳

MEDICATION Pigmentation may be induced by a wide variety of drugs including nonsteroidal anti-inflammatory drugs like ibuprofen.

Anti-acne drugs like tetracycline and doxycycline are also a problem.

TOPICAL ANTIMICROBIALS Topical antibacterial acne medication like benzoyl peroxide creates free radicals that cause inflammation leading to hyperpigmentation.

HYDROQUINONE This strong skin-bleaching agent is linked to cancer and banned in Europe and Asia.

CHEMICAL SUNSCREENS Ingredients like oxybenzone, octinoxate, octocrylene and avobenzone break down in the presence of UV to produce free radicals.

FRAGRANCES Perfumed alcohol or photosensitizing essential oils like bergamot can cause hyperpigmentation in areas where it is frequently applied.

RESOURCES

1. PubMed.gov, J Invest Dermatol. 2010 Dec; 130(12):2719-26. doi: 10.1038/jid.2010.204. Epub 2010 Jul 22. Airborne particle exposure and extrinsic skin aging.

THE FUTURE
of SKIN CARE

· SECTION ·
THREE

SKIN MICROBIOME RESEARCH

FASHIONABLE NOTIONS OF BEAUTY COME AND GO. The Ruben-esque form with luscious curves lolling on a canopied bed gives way to a skeletal model teetering down a run-way on six-inch stilettos. But regardless of *la mode du jour*, beautiful skin is always in.

CLEAR, RADIANT SKIN HAS SEEMED UNATTAINABLE for too many people for too long, but thanks to advancements in science, with skin microbiome research leading the way, achieving that impossible dream is closer than ever.

WHAT STARTS in the GUT...

One theory of ill health is that most problems begin with microbial imbalances in the gut. More specifically, problems start with the lining of the digestive tract, called the epithelium. The surface area of this internal skin, large enough to cover a tennis court, mediates our relationship to the world outside our bodies; more than 50 tons of food pass through it in a lifetime. The microbiota play a critical role in maintaining the health of the epithelium, including bacteria, like the *bifidobacteria* and *Lactobacillus plantarum* found in fermented vegetables.

The epithelium, unlike most tissues, does not get its nourishment from the bloodstream, but from short-chain fatty acids produced by gut bacteria as a byproduct of their fermentation of plant fiber in the large intestine.

The epithelial barrier, when insufficiently nourished, becomes less efficient at preventing bacteria and byproducts of certain bacteria (endotoxins) from reaching the bloodstream. When this happens the body's immune system goes into action, resulting in low-grade inflammation that can affect the entire body.

GOES to the SKIN...

It's easy to see parallels between the gut epithelium and the largest organ of the human body when acting as barriers protecting against surrounding elements. The external skin, though not as large as a tennis court but still substantial at 1.5 to 2.0 square meters, has other vital functions less clearly understood. Until recently the preponderance of studies has focused on how microorganisms in the gut regulate the immune system and inflammation. Now, a new paper published in *Science*[1] shows us definitively that skin has a parallel immunological response to that seen in the gut.

Indeed, as it turns out, skin flora can drive local immunity in a way that is not replicated by the gut. For example, germ-free mice were unable to mount an immune response to the pathogen *Leishmania major*. When *Staphylococcus epidermidis*, a common skin commensal, was reintroduced to the skin it was enough to reinstate the production of an inflammatory protein by T-cells in the skin—but not in the gut.

"THE GUT MICROBIOME HAS BEEN THE FOCUS FOR THE LAST TEN YEARS—NOW IT'S THE SKIN'S TURN."
— SKIN MICROBIOME-RESEARCHER JULIE SEGRE
Study Co-Author, National Human Genome Research Institute, Bethesda, MD

BEYOND to the CLOUD...

The residents of the gut, and respiratory, oral and vaginal microbiomes are mostly inside dwellers. But when we zero in on the skin, the housing structures change. First, the folds, follicles and tiny oil-producing glands on the skin's surface create a multitude of diverse habitats, each with its own community.

The microorganisms living on the surface also create a cloud that surrounds us and could be seen if we had microvision. So it's no surprise that each of us supports a 'microcloud' all our own.

An individual's microorganisms are a product of that particular host's genetics and environment—what she eats, where she lives and what she puts on her skin.

...and BACK to the FUTURE

This microbiome uniqueness introduces exciting prospects for treating stubborn skin conditions that persist, no matter what we do. Long-standing acne is a perfect case in point.

THE C. DIFFICILE STORY *Clostridium difficile* is a bacterium that causes diarrhea and more serious intestinal conditions such as colitis. Increasing in incidence, severity and mortality, treatments with antibiotics like vancomycin have been discouraging. Vancomycin supports the fact that antibiotic treatment can be extensive, expensive and, ultimately, ineffective.

The increasing problems accompanying conventional therapy helps explain the growing acceptance of a new treatment protocol that sounds off-putting at first. The treatment is called fecal microbiota transplantation (FMT), and according to case studies[2] about 90% of patients who undergo it are cured for good.

THE FUTURE OF SKIN CARE

Antibiotics were a life-saving discovery unlike any other and medicine's guiding light throughout the 20th century. The *C. diff* success story is the first indication of how microbiome research is starting to transform 21st-century medical thinking.

It's an exciting time to be in research—and soon it will be the skin's turn to enjoy improved treatment outcomes by way of innovative findings.

~~~~~~

HAPPY MICROBES = HAPPY SKIN

Recent work sheds more light on the critical role played by microbiota in maintaining skin health. Some bacteria, like *P. acnes*, produce the short chain fatty acids that regulate lubrication, maintain barrier function and keep pathogens at bay.

Part of the canon of acne treatments has always been that *P. acnes* is the main culprit contributing to acne, and in 20th-century thinking it made sense that once you destroy the microbe you cure the problem. Thus benzoyl peroxide (BP), the powerful antimicrobial, charged in to save the day.

It's true that short-term gains are often made using BP, but the long-term effects—diminished efficacy, photosensitization and premature skin aging—make the BP vs. *P. acnes* tale sound like a dismal repeat of the oral vancomycin vs. *C. diff* story—it works (with downsides) until it doesn't.

You can see the dilemma—*P. acnes* is needed to maintain active lipid metabolism, but in some cases it causes acne. Fortunately our 21st-century researchers are hard at work, discovering new, alternative forms of treatment.

~~~~~~

GOOD vs. BAD MICROBES

We have reached the research point where we can start to identify which microbes may act to maintain microbial equilibrium. Potential candidates are:

STAPHYLOCOCCUS EPIDERMIDIS—this commensal produces succinic acid, which has been shown to inhibit *P. acnes* growth.

LACTOBACILLIS PLANTARUM has anti-inflammatory properties and appears to reduce the size of acne lesions when applied topically.

This study[3] suggests a novel approach to an old problem.

"Metagenomic analysis demonstrated that although the relative abundances of *P. acnes* were similar, the strain population structures were significantly different in the two cohorts. Certain strains were highly associated with acne, and other strains were enriched in healthy skin. By sequencing 66 previously unreported *P. acnes* strains and comparing 71 *P. acnes* genomes, we identified potential genetic determinants of various *P. acnes* strains in association with acne or health."

"Our analysis suggests that acquired DNA sequences and bacterial immune elements may have roles in determining virulence properties of *P. acnes* strains, and some could be future targets for therapeutic interventions. This study demonstrates a previously unreported paradigm of commensal strain populations that could explain the pathogenesis of human diseases. It underscores the importance of strain-level analysis of the human microbiome to define the role of commensals in health and disease."

In short, everyone harbors *P. acnes*. Commensal bacteria serve a crucial role in maintaining healthy skin. People who develop acne may have virulent strains of *P. acnes* not found in healthy skins.

A 21st-century approach to resolving acne involves taking a promicrobial rather than an antimicrobial stance. Instead of annihilating all *P. acnes*, with its concomitant detrimental consequences to skin health, why not transplant healthy strains of *P. acnes* to people who harbor virulent strains?

TAKING THE LEAP:
20th into 21st CENTURY

We know that nourishing the gut prevents microbial imbalances that could result in chronic inflammation. The next step is to carry that same thinking to skin care. Unfortunately, most of the advice we receive is still firmly mired in the 20th century. Follow the chart below to see if you've made the temporal leap. If you haven't, take heart—it's easier than you think. Welcome to the 21st!

NOTE TO ADULT ACNE SUFFERERS for the following 20th to 21st-century treatment reference (pg. 154-159):

● = TREATMENTS THAT CAN CAUSE PREMATURE AGING

● = TREATMENTS THAT CAN DELAY AGING

RESOURCES:

1. Nature News: The skin's secret surveillance system by Virginia Gewin, July 26, 2012, Copyright © 2012, Rights Managed by Nature Publishing Group

2. Clin Gastroenterol Hepatol. Treating Clostridium difficile Infection with Fecal Microbiota Transplantation, Author manuscript; available in PMC 2012 Dec 1. Published in final edited form as: Clin Gastroenterol Hepatol. 2011 Dec; 9(12): 1044—1049. Published online 2011 Aug 24. doi: 10.1016/j.cgh.2011.08.014 PMCID: PMC3223289 NIHMSID: NIHMS320727

3. PubMed: J Invest Dermatol. Propionibacterium acnes strain populations in the human skin microbiome associated with acne. 2013 Sep;133(9):2152-60. doi: 10.1038/jid.2013.21. Epub 2013 Jan 21.

20th-CENTURY TREATMENTS	EXAMPLES / THERAPEUTIC RATIONALE	RESULT or POSSIBLE OUTCOMES
OIL-FREE MOISTURIZERS	Moisturizers with silicone, dimethicone / Oil was thought to clog pores	Skin becomes drier, more congestion occurs
EXFOLIATION WITH SCRUBS	Apricot kernel scrub / Exfoliation of dead skin cells to unclog pores	Causes microscopic tears, providing entry for harmful bacteria
EXFOLIATION WITH ALPHA HYDROXY ACIDS (AHAS) / BETA HYDROXY ACIDS (BHAS)	Peels remove layers of dead skin cells, increase cell turnover rate	AHAs: Glycolic acid, Malic acid, Tartaric acid. May cause skin irritation w/ overuse; hyperpigmentation may develop in ethnic skin, especially Asian, African

21st-CENTURY TREATMENTS	EXAMPLES / THERAPEUTIC RATIONALE	RESULT or POSSIBLE OUTCOMES
TOPICAL OILS WITH OMEGA 3-6 BALANCE	Krill oil, kiwi seed, flax seed, etc. / Oils improve barrier function and dissolve congestion below the surface	Less congestion, less acne formation, reduced inflammation, strengthened stratum corneum, age-delaying effects
EXFOLIATION WITH OILS	Olive oil, sunflower oil, etc. Removes dead skin cells without tearing skin	Deeper cleansing of pores, improved barrier function
EXFOLIATION WITH SELECT HYDROXY ACIDS	Salicylic acid (a BHA), Lactic acid (an AHA)	Salicylic acid dissolves skin protein from the outside, unclogs pores. Lactic acid increases cell turnover rate.

● = TREATMENT CAN DELAY AGING

20th-CENTURY TREATMENTS	EXAMPLES / THERAPEUTIC RATIONALE	RESULT or POSSIBLE OUTCOMES
ANTIBIOTICS	Tetracycline, erythromycin / Kill microbial populations that cause acne	Antibiotic resistance may develop. Microbiome becomes out of balance, leading to inflammation.
ANTIANDROGEN THERAPY	Spironolactone Cyproterone acetate / Reduces adrenal androgen production; counteracts effect of testosterone on skin	Often successful in cases of polycystic ovary syndrome (PCOS) Skin reverts when meds are discontinued; physical side effects include nausea, fatigue and headaches

21st-CENTURY TREATMENTS	EXAMPLES / THERAPEUTIC RATIONALE	RESULT or POSSIBLE OUTCOMES
PROBIOTICS	Yogurt and fermented foods Balance gut and skin microbiomes	Bolster immune system, reduce inflammation
VITAMINS AND MINERALS	B5 and B3, zinc, calcium/ magnesium, krill oil / B5 produces Coenzyme-A to break down sebum. B3 and omega 3s reduce inflammation and acne associated with zinc/mineral deficiencies	Gradual improvement of acne without side effects such as premature aging or systemic disruptions leading to future health problems

● = TREATMENT CAN DELAY AGING

20th-CENTURY TREATMENTS	EXAMPLES / THERAPEUTIC RATIONALE	RESULT or POSSIBLE OUTCOMES
TOPICAL ANTIMICROBIALS	Benzoyl peroxide, Triclosan / Target *P. acnes*	Increased sun sensitivity, Premature aging
ISOTRETINOIN	Accutane / Shrinks sebaceous glands, Reduces sebum production	Good success rate, but side effects such as skin irritation, rashes, extreme dryness and depression range from moderate to severe
BLUE LIGHT THERAPY	LED (light emitting diode) treatments / Kills *P. acnes* by creating oxygen-free radicals	Possible inflammation or skin burning, Premature aging

21st-CENTURY TREATMENTS	EXAMPLES / THERAPEUTIC RATIONALE	RESULT or POSSIBLE OUTCOMES
MICROBIAL BOOSTERS	*S. epidermidis* *Lactobacillus plantarum* *S. thermophilus*	Aid skin's immune system response, improve barrier function. *S. thermophilis* may have age-delaying effects
RETIN A / RETINOL	Regulate sebum, Normalize skin cell development, Reduce inflammation	Normalizes sebum production without negative side effects Age-delaying: boosts collagen production and reverses photodamage
MICROBIAL TRANSPLANTS	Replenish skin with "missing microbes" contributing to skin health	Potential solution for skin disorders with resistantance to conventional therapies, like acne and eczema

● = TREATMENT CAN DELAY AGING

EPIGENETICS: THE MISSING MICRONUTRIENTS

DR. MARTIN BLASER PENNED THE GROUNDBREAKING WORK, "THE MISSING MICROBES," which describes how antibiotic overuse slaughters "good" microbes along with the "bad" to the detriment of our health. In the absence of certain hardworking microbes we cannot digest our food or frankly, do much of anything.

Now epigenetic research is joining microbiome research as another discipline set to overturn our worldview when it comes to disease. Think of genes as the hardware and the epigenome as the software that controls your genes' on/off switch.

Epigenetics explains how heritable changes in genome function are influenced by factors like environment, diet and lifestyle—without changing DNA sequence. In other words, you can't change your DNA, but you can affect the way it behaves.

IS ACNE INHERITED?

"My father had terrible skin, and I am the sibling who inherited it. My sister and my brother both have perfect skin."

I hear variations on this story all the time, and the answer is: Yes, you may inherit a tendency to acne or even have acne, but you're not hopelessly doomed by your genetics.

Epigenetic research shows us how micronutrient deficiency contributes to disorders we always thought of as being "inherited," or an ineradicable part of our DNA code. Although the genetics-is-destiny mantra holds true to a large extent, epigenetics research illuminates ways in which we, often unwittingly, are in the process of modulating inherited traits via what we eat, as well as a host of other lifestyle factors.

In a fascinating study[1], brown-coated male and female agouti mice produced strawberry blond offspring when the mother was fed a folic acid-deficient diet. Zoe Draelos, M.D., consulting professor, Department of Dermatology, Duke University School of Medicine, points out that, "Not only does the baby have strawberry blonde hair, but that genetic line is changed from that point forward. The offspring of that mouse will also have a gene for strawberry blond hair—even though its grandparents had no such gene."

She goes on to suggest that the agouti mouse experiment is behind the emerging importance of micronutrients in the study of skin. Micronutrients are substances that, though necessary only in very tiny amounts, are nevertheless integral in maintaining health and delaying premature aging.

Most of us may be aware of the value of folic acid for proper fetal development, but we remain blissfully unaware of the need for other micronutrients, including minerals and trace minerals. Sadly, most of us are woefully deficient in minerals and trace minerals formerly found in topsoil and incorporated into plants, because industrial farming methods have virtually wiped them out. Adding insult to injury, we drink bottled water or filtered water depleted of its mineral content. Many micronutrient deficiencies first show in the skin. Along with type 2 diabetes and cancer, epigenetic changes have been identified in skin disorders such as:

→ PSORIASIS
(Zhang P, Su Y, Lu Q. J Eur Acad Dermatol Venereol. 2012;26(4):399-403)

→ MELANOMA
(Patino WD, Susa J. Adv Dermatol. 2008;24:59- 70. Review)

→ SYSTEMIC LUPUS ERYTHEMATOSUS
(Millington GW. Pharmacogenomics. 2008;9(12):1835-1850)

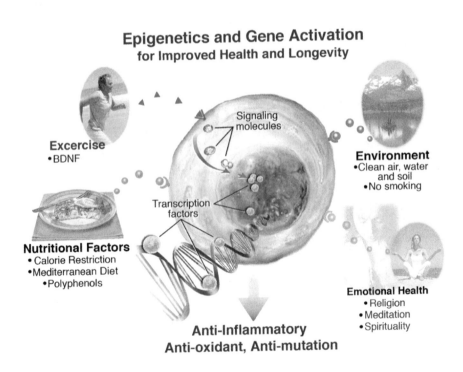

Epigenetics and Gene Activation
for Improved Health and Longevity

Excercise
•BDNF

Signaling molecules

Transcription factors

Environment
•Clean air, water and soil
•No smoking

Nutritional Factors
• Calorie Restriction
•Mediterranean Diet
•Polyphenols

Emotional Health
• Religion
• Meditation
•Spirituality

Anti-Inflammatory
Anti-oxidant, Anti-mutation

©2009 JOSEPH MAROON, MD

The concept of epigenetic influences from outside the cell sources (exercise, nutrition, environment and emotion) that can activate nuclear transcription factors that can result in either very healthy (anti-inflammatory, antioxidant, anti-mutation) or unhealthy conditions being propagated from DNA codes.

THE FUTURE OF SKIN CARE

WHICH MICRONUTRIENTS
✳ FOR ACNE ✳

We've discussed some nutrients, vitamin B5 for example, whose absence has significant impact on acne development. Antioxidant vitamins C and E are vastly important in maintaining skin health, but so is the micronutrient selenium, which works in an antioxidant pathway completely separate from vitamins C and E. Selenium provides oxidative protection indispensible in preventing skin cancers and other oxidative insults to the body.

Read on for mineral micronutrients that have proven to make an impressive difference in the acne battle. Minerals that can be taken internally as well as applied topically include:

ZINC Many studies indicate that acne sufferers tend to be zinc-deficient.

→ INTERNAL / 1 x DAY
   Zinc methionine and zinc gluconate are easily absorbed.

→ EXTERNAL / DAILY
   Using a daily sunscreen high in zinc oxide is another way to get your zinc, as well as protect against UV damage.

MAGNESIUM is required for over 300 enzymes to function properly. The recommended daily nutritional requirement of the mineral is 300-400 mg.

INTERNALLY: MAGNESIUM CITRATE To improve the absorption of magnesium, it is recommended that vitamin C and calcium supplements be taken with magnesium.

EXTERNALLY: MAGNESIUM CHLORIDE or MAGNESIUM SULFATE (aka Epsom salts) is highly anti-inflammatory and often used to hasten healing of surface wounds. It can be sprayed on the skin or used in the tub.

ADDITIONAL MICRONUTRIENTS

SELENIUM deficiency can contribute to acne woes, bur it is possible to take too much; avoid overdoing supplementation. Just two Brazil nuts a day will provide you with plenty of selenium. Other food sources include egg yolks, meat and fish.

COPPER is a tricky one, since minerals in your body are often matched in ratios with their 'partner minerals.' Copper competes with zinc in the body, so if you're not getting enough zinc or your body is using it up too fast, copper levels may increase.

If your body retains too much copper, it can deplete your zinc. If you suspect your acne may be caused by a zinc deficiency related to copper toxicity, consider investing in a hair analysis. The results will tell you if you need to increase your zinc.

TRACE MINERALS

The minerals above are the tip of the iceberg. The ocean supplies >70 different elements and minerals that we need. Without them, we risk a significant effect on our health. Like microbes, their absence could lead to problems.

HOW WILL YOU KNOW...

MISSING SOMETHING? Women and men deficient in minerals (about 90% of the population according to some experts) due to stress, frequent exercise or a micronutrient-poor diet might experience muscle cramps, food cravings or general fatigue. Another tip-off is skin problems like acne, psoriasis or eczema.

WHAT'S MISSING? Humans are estimated to need about two-thirds of the known elements. Considering that there are 92 known elements, 22 waiting verification and hundreds of isotopes, we can assume that something is missing. This is particularly true the farther we are from the ocean—the primal source of most of these minerals.

IN WHAT AMOUNTS? The safest source of mineral supplementation is the ocean. And, since they're predetermined by nature, you can't go wrong with the proportions.

HOW TO GET THEM? Take minerals and trace minerals internally daily. If you're concerned about ingesting too much internally, spraying them on the skin is a refreshing alternative. Transdermal delivery is especially recommended in cases where skin problems related to micronutrient deficiency have been identified. A spray increases bioavailability of the micronutrients to the organ in need by directly targeting the tissue with minerals that are water soluble and readily absorbed.

RESOURCES

1. Dermatology Times: Micronutrients may play role in skincare and dermatologic diseases by John Jesitus, April 01, 2013

THE HOLISTIC APPROACH: AN INTERVIEW WITH KRISTINA HOLEY

NEW CHANGES IN PRODUCT DEVELOPMENT ARE IMMINENT AS WE BROADEN OUR VIEW OF SKIN to include, as well as the dermis, epidermis and stratum corneum, the fourth unseen layer—the skin microbiome. Microorganisms live on the skin's surface, in eyebrows and lashes, in deeper layers of the skin, hair follicles and sebaceous glands.

Many of these same microorganisms are also found in our oral and respiratory microbiomes, and above all, in the gut. To be accurate, we should call the gut-brain axis, the gut/brain/skin axis, for all micro-life is connected. We're just beginning to recognize the depth and inseparability of these connections.

Our new understanding will profoundly alter the ways in which practitioners deliver skin care.

IMPORTANT CHANGES
NOW GLIMMER on OUR HORIZON

INSTANT GRATIFICATION DEMAND SUBSIDES thanks to unforeseen and unpleasant consequences that so often accompany the quick fix.

LESS RELIANCE ON GIMMICKS like epidermal planing, light treatments and deep-cleansing devices that abrade the skin, compromise barrier protection and disrupt microbial communities—all of which pave the way for infection.

EDUCATION AS THE BACKBONE OF TREATMENT Practitioners will understand the reasoning and research behind their preferred products and treatments.

TREATMENTS CUSTOMIZED TO THE INDIVIDUAL Holistic methods involving comprehensive studies addressing all aspects of the whole body will replace fountain-of-youth promises and bogus gizmos.

PRACTITIONER/CLIENT RELATIONSHIP = TREATMENT SUCCESS On the practitioner's side will come a commitment to using knowledge to provide long-term and permanent improvement—without promising a quick fix or miracle cure. On the client's side will come a commitment to adopting necessary lifestyle changes, and most importantly, patience and trust.

One lesson we've learned is that successfully treating acne or premature skin aging isn't a matter of taking a pill, slathering on a lotion, fixing digestive problems or improving your diet. Doing all those things can help, but only with the proper guidance. The right skin care practitioner can make all the difference.

The good news is such people do exist.

MEET KRISTINA HOLEY

KRISTINA HOLEY comes to skin care via a route familiar to many of us who end up, often circuitously, in the skin care business. It begins with a personal story about misbehaving skin. Kristina was diagnosed with polycystic ovary syndrome (PCOS) in her teens and, though in keeping with her symptoms, was unsupported by diagnostic tests. Her frustration with that diagnosis led to a lifelong quest to find better answers. Fortunately Kristina's surgeon father encouraged a spirit of skeptical inquiry, but rather than going to medical school as originally planned, she went in a different direction. Her quest to learn about all things skin-related led her to Paris, where she studied at the Institut Superieur International des Parfums (ISIPCA) under the auspices of world-renowned biochemist Joëlle Ciocco.

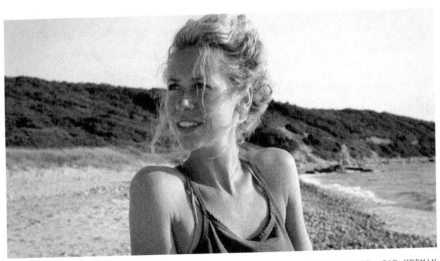

PHOTO CREDIT: GAB HERMAN

THE FUTURE OF SKIN CARE

In the process of diagnosing what was really going on with her own skin, she discovered her passion for skin-detective work on a grand scale. Finding the patterns that inform skin problems, especially the most challenging, guided her through years of intensive study. Over time Kristina's extensive knowledge combined with her ability to observe keenly and follow a logical trail, led to stardom in the skin care world equivalent to Sherlock's status amongst detectives. With persistence, intelligence, imagination and guts, Kristina can arrive at conclusions hidden to most people.

A-list clients consult her regularly, and without naming names (you'd recognize them instantly...), we included a few enlightening histories from her case files.

CLIENT #1: KALINDA, AGE 31

FIRST IMPRESSIONS When I met Kalinda she had "good skin," that is, absent of obvious problems, but it was dry, imbalanced and the cheek region was full of "dormant" congestion with rough and uneven texture. The overall tone was dull and splotchy. There seemed to be fluid retention and congestion inhibiting free lymph flow contributing to the lack of brightness in skin tone.

HEALTH Kalinda complained of not feeling well most of the time. She was extremely constipated, had monthly recurrence of UTIs that were treated with antibiotics every month, and very irregular eating patterns due to extreme GI discomfort.

TREATMENT PROGRAM My priority was to balance the skin's ecosystem from a bacterial level. In addition to putting her on a low-inflammatory diet for a month, consisting of mostly cooked foods to be eaten at regular intervals, I encouraged her to visit an acupuncturist for digestive help.

Her digestion shifted very quickly and soon she was no longer constipated. However her congested cheek region became full of deep, cystic pimples.

The more stimulated her digestion was, the more she began to break out. This continued for a few months, with never really severe acne, but consistently one or two cysts at a time.

We followed regular acupuncture and enzymes with probiotics and a strategic diet, and while she was feeling really good her skin was purging pretty much all the time. The internal cleansing and rebuilding went on for six months, and during that time her skin really suffered. The oil levels fluctuated, as did the inflammation.

TOPICAL TREATMENTS In the midst of her digestive rehab she was also changing her skin care routine to include a lot of stimulation.

Her moisturizer was a blend of black cumin oil and jojoba, which she massaged into her skin, cleansing afterwards with a salicylic acid wash three times a week.

The daily massage with cumin and jojoba was meant to be deep and to stimulate all areas of the face. The biggest shift here was the swelling around the eyes. Every morning she woke up with puffy lower lids, but after massaging the eye contour region on a regular basis the swelling diminished and finally cleared. On the rare occasions she did wake up with swelling, it cleared quickly with a little massage.

Besides the oil massages she kept it simple with weekly yogurt masks. She treated breakouts with a mask made of clay, zinc, sulfur and tea tree oil—egg whites also really helped. To treat a single pimple she'd use pure zinc or pure sulfur to which she added drop of water to make a paste.

OUTCOME After six months her skin was clear. Now, a year later, she has no breakouts whatsoever, and her skin is really healthy, glowing and oil-rich (seriously!).

Her current product list is minimal: a cleanser, an oil blend and retinol at night.

CLIENT #2: SOPHIE, AGE 43

FIRST IMPRESSIONS Sophie was a classic example of what can happen when you overdo it. When I first saw her she was on 0.1% Retin A daily, and using a benzoyl peroxide wash delivered via a sonic cleansing device twice a day. No surprise that her skin was red, highly inflamed and deeply dehydrated, with cystic acne along the cheeks.

In contrast to most hormonal acne where areas affected include jaw line and forehead, her acne was entirely concentrated on her cheeks between the jaw and cheekbone. There was a greasy texture to the skin, rather than oily, and the epidermal layer felt completely "closed." I see this often when cases of adolescent acne merge into adult acne without ever being corrected.

It appeared to be a case of chronic acne starting at puberty, in which all the triggering factors were in play: excess sebum production, pore congestion leading to over-colonization of *P. acnes* and subsequent inflammation.

HEALTH Sophie, mother of two, had a long history of constipation, mix-managed blood sugar, years of birth control and chronic adult acne. She has been under a dermatologist's care and has had Accutane treatments twice over the past fifteen years.

TREATMENT PROGRAM The first order of business was to stimulate her digestion, which was seriously under par and contributed to many of her problems. The focus was on getting her to have regular bowel movements via strategic and structured eating, enzymes and probiotics. At the same time I had her increase her vitamin B intake, especially vitamin B5, through diet and supplements.

TOPICAL TREATMENTS The goal was to gradually wean her away from prescription products, switching from Retin-A to retinol for example, followed by a vitamin B5 serum to regulate sebum production, and an oil blend containing bioflavonoids and tea tree essential oil to replace benzoyl peroxide in order to control *P. acnes* overgrowth.

We also changed up her cleansing routine, going from BP washes with a sonic cleaner twice daily to once daily, at night, using a gentle cleanser and no sonic cleaner. Mornings she could use tepid water. The weaning process took approximately one month.

OUTCOME The results were actually very fast. After one skin cycle, her skin was open, hydrated, soothed and actually looked "alive." The quality of her skin shifted from a lifeless, barren desert to renewed healthy skin—dramatically less greasy, red and inflamed. Some breakouts continued, but were far less frequent. One year later they are a rare occurrence.

She is still juggling her stress, eating habits and healing from years and years of constipation, which probably accounts for the leftover cheek pimples that occasionally pop up. The quality of her skin, however, is night and day—to the point where she doesn't even mind the occasional breakout. The scarring is healing and the overall skin tone is much brighter and clearer.

CLIENT #3: ZOE, AGE 33

FIRST IMPRESSIONS Zoe represents a type of client I see frequently in my urban practice: young, active, combining lots of high-intensity exercise with raw/cold food fad diets on the extreme side (think smoothies, salads, sushi, granola/yogurt, juices). The high-anxiety levels exacerbated by her lifestyle were not relieved by sleep, which was sporadic and not restful.

Her skin was imbalanced with areas of dryness and oiliness intermixed. She had mild perioral dermatitis, presented as redness in the chin, nose and mouth areas, and in addition, she had redness between the eyes. She would experience breakouts in the center of her chin, one pimple on either side of her chin at ovulation, and a few days before her period, inflammation around the ears, hairline and jawline, resulting in one or two pimples.

HEALTH Zoe suffered from quite a few symptoms common to high-performing, high-anxiety people. The sleep deficit she'd built up over years was not alleviated by intense exercise; in fact too much exercise was making restful sleep less attainable. She was also struggling to control bouts of loose bowels and moderately spiking blood sugar levels with diet.

TREATMENT PROGRAM The treatment program I designed for Zoe addressed two factors: first and most important, the chronic inflammation resulting from years of microbial imbalances and subsequent digestive problems; second, the hormonal breakouts occurring at pre-period and at ovulation. The program would focus on altering both her external and internal environments, which meant changing both her diet and skin care routines.

INTERNAL

№ 1 EAT A DIET OF COOKED FOODS not too high in fiber or fruit, low in sugar, high in protein and complex carbs. Keep blood sugar levels on an even keel by drinking plenty of water and, as much as possible, by avoiding foods contributing to inflammation such as gluten, dairy, sugar, alcohol, caffeine, corn, soy, processed foods and so on. Include foods high in B vitamins, selenium, manganese, omega 3s and fatty proteins at all times, and especially during stages of the monthly cycle when most prone to breakouts.

→ ALL MONTH
Lots of dark leafy greens (preferably cooked), animal proteins, eggs and good fats

→ RIGHT AFTER YOU FINISH BLEEDING
Oats, artichoke, broccoli, carrots, parsley, beans, zucchini

→ RIGHT BEFORE YOU START BLEEDING
Brown rice, millet, cauliflower, collards, onion, daikon, parsnip, radish, sweet potato

→ WHILE BLEEDING
Beets, kale, kelp, mushrooms, buckwheat

№ 2 MODERATE HIGH-INTENSITY EXERCISE Okay around ovulation, minimize around period, focus on plenty of sleep throughout the month, and stress management.

№ 3 SUPPLEMENTS Alternate months with probiotics and include cultured foods at onset of largest meal. Take vitamin B-Complex, 250 mgs B5, omega-3 fish oil and astaxanthin daily. Soak in Epsom salt baths three times a week for the magnesium.

EXTERNAL

While I felt that Zoe's breakouts were nearly 100% caused by inflammation related to her digestive problems and hormonal imbalances, her skin care routine certainly left much to be desired. Because Zoe was just as inclined to follow the latest skin care fad as the latest dietary one, she was constantly changing products—going from oil blends with high levels of essential oils to stripping salicylic acid cleansers and spot treatments, then using thick creams when her skin felt extra dry.

What her skin craved was a regular skin care routine without the extremes. To wean her from her excesses, binge feeding her skin oils and creams one day, then "purging" it the next with acid washes, we replaced all her products with mild, non-invasive ones she could use every day. All of them were designed to nourish her skin without stressing it.

MY SUGGESTIONS

№ 1 IN PLACE OF STRIPPING CLEANSERS Use a cleanser that cleans skin gently without raising pH levels. Cleanse once a day, at night.

№ 2 USE HOMEMADE RINSES after cleansing, like a diluted apple cider vinegar or green tea/nettle tea.

№ 3 AVOID OIL BLENDS WITH TOO MANY ESSENTIAL OILS I suspected that the essential oils contributed to her perioral dermatitis, since many EO's cause allergic dermatitis. Substitute oils high in EFAs and saturated fats to improve barrier function.

№ 4 APPLY RETINOL AT NIGHT to regulate turnover rate, keep pores clear and minimize inflammation.

№ 5 USE ZINC-BASED SUNSCREEN DAILY

№ 6 MASKS included a goat milk yogurt/manuka honey/spirulina mask, and every two weeks a lactic acid/enzyme mask to exfoliate.

OUTCOME The protocol has been in action a little over a year and the chin breakouts are now 99% eliminated, as are the hormonal breakouts at ovulation and pre-period.

I attribute the main cause of success to a better diet, both internally and externally. Healthy food, regular (not excessive) exercise and clean skin care products were key to reducing the inflammation that was the root cause of her skin problems.

USAGE AND RESOURCE GUIDE

№ 1 THE DIY ADVANTAGE (177)

The freshest products are those you prepare at home. You can make them in small batches, store them in your refrigerator—and save money. Your local grocery store is likely to carry all the ingredients you'll need.

№ 2 SPECIALTY ITEMS & FINISHED PRODUCTS (185)

Specialty items not readily made at home, like salicylic acid cleansers, alpha and beta hydroxy lotions or retinol/retinaldehyde serums, can be immensely helpful in clearing acne. This guide includes product recommendations and where they can be purchased, with options to fit every budget.

№ 3 SAMPLE AM/PM ROUTINES USING REAL PRODUCTS (196)

I modeled these routines on our successful case study, Clara. Initially I resisted this approach because her regimen included Marie Veronique products exclusively, and I want my readers to know that there are other products I trust to work just as well. The products listed in this guide are based on the admiration I have for companies who confront the complexities of safe and effective formulation with integrity and success. I know from experience that this is not easily accomplished.

But neither is the task of making your skin healthier or sleuthing out the best way to help your teenage son or daughter deal with acne, so in the spirit of simplicity, I offer up sample routines. Please feel free to adapt or modify them according to your needs. Each of us is different, no two skins are the same, and every skin micro-biome is unique. The important thing in the midst of all this differentness is to find out what works for you.

№ 1 DIY SOLUTIONS

Using ingredients commonly found in grocery stores, supermarkets and/or natural foods store.

CLEANSING, MOISTURIZING & EXFOLIATING

YOGURT

Good for all skin types; especially for rosacea-prone, sensitive and mature skin. Suggested uses:

CLEANSER Spread ½ tsp yogurt over face, cleanse with tepid water.

MOISTURIZER Put ¼ tsp on cleansed skin, leave on overnight, wash off with tepid water the next day.

EXFOLIATOR Put ½ tsp yogurt on cleansed face and neck, leave on 15 -20 minutes, rinse with warm water.

→ WHAT TO BUY
Organic full-fat yogurt, plain. Goat or sheep yogurts work well. Live, active cultures, especially *S. Thermophilus, L. Bulgaricus, L. Acidophilus, Bifidus and L. Casei,* included in the list of ingredients. Organic full-fat

yogurt, plain. Goat or sheep yogurts work well. If you are allergic to dairy, try soy-based or coconut-based yogurts.

→ SUGGESTED BRANDS
Greek Gods, Noosa (from Australia)

→ WHERE TO BUY
Grocery stores and supermarkets.

OILS HIGH IN ESSENTIAL FATTY ACIDS
(Especially omega 6 and omega 3)

Good for all skin types, but especially dry, mature skin or skin with a lot of congestion, i.e., blackheads and whiteheads. Suggested uses:

CLEANSER Simply massage about ½ tsp onto face, then either rinse or wipe off. Olive oil is good for dry skin, sunflower, safflower or grapeseed oils are good if your skin is oily or congested.

MOISTURIZER Apply ½ tsp to damp or dry skin of face and neck, leave on. If your skin is dry, a mix of omega 3s to omega 6s, for example ¼ cup walnut seed oil to ¼ cup sunflower oil, is fine. Massage into cleansed skin and leave on overnight.

EXFOLIATOR TO CLEAR CONGESTION See Exfoliation section below.

→ WHAT TO BUY
Cold-pressed, unrefined oils.

Oils high in omega 3: flaxseed, hempseed and walnut oils are helpful if your skin is mature dry and inflamed.

Oils high in omega 6: safflower, sunflower and grapeseed oils thin out dense, thick sebum, so it can travel through pores to lubricate the surface of the skin.

→ IF YOU HAVE DRY SKIN
Omega 3-to-6 ratio can be 1-to-1.

→ IF YOU HAVE OILY & CONGESTED SKIN
Use omega 6 to omega 3 in a ratio of 2 parts safflower oil (or
other omega 6) to 1 part flaxseed oil (or other omega 3).

OTHER OILS

TEA TREE OIL an essential oil. Look for 100% tea tree oil from the Melaleuca alternifotia tree. (Over 100 different types of Melaleuca exist, and many
are used for their oils.) To guarantee quality and purity, the label should identify the oil as, "100% Australian tea tree oil from the Melaleuca alternifotia
tree" along with a "T" value on the label.

COCONUT OIL / SPECIAL NOTE Despite its many proponents coconut
oil is on my "avoid list" for anyone with acne. It can be highly comedogenic for
some people, and if you fall into that category it could take awhile to recover
from flare-ups.

It also contains no essential fatty acids, which are what skin, like the rest of
your body, need in daily doses. As a moisturizer for your body or as a hair
treatment coconut oil is fine, just avoid using it on face and neck, or anywhere
you break out.

→ SUGGESTED BRANDS
Spectrum is a good organic brand with many oil choices. For tea tree oil,
try Humco or Desert Essence.

→ WHERE TO BUY
All can be purchased at grocery stores and supermarkets. Find tea tree
oil brands, Humco and Desert Essence, in drug stores.

HYDRATION & TONING

GREEN TEA

(Anti-Inflammatory, anti-acne, UV protection booster)

Good for all skin types, safe even for babies. Especially good for skins prone to inflammation; also has great anti-acne properties. Excellent for soothing sun-exposed skin. Suggested uses:

DAILY HYDRATION for all skin types: After cleansing, mist on green tea. Continue with applications of your morning and nightly serums and oils while face is still damp.

ANTI-INFLAMMATORY / ANTI-ACNE Take your spray bottle for use after sports when you've been sweating or have gotten overheated. If you can't shower, splash on warm water, then mist with your spray. Use as often as desired.

PROTECTION BOOST Green tea has some UV-filtering capabilities. Use to boost your sunscreen protection and to cool off on hot days. Take a spray bottle to the beach, on hikes and sports events (either watching or participating).

DIY RECIPE Pour 3 to 4 cups boiling water over three to five teabags. Let steep ½ hour. Remove teabags, refrigerate, then pour into a spray bottle when cooled. Keep refrigerated. You may add ¼ tsp licorice root extract if you have trouble with inflammation.

→ WHAT TO BUY
Green tea bags or loose tea. Organic is good, but not necessary.

Choose the tea highest in epigallo-catechin gallate (ECGC). In a study, green tea bags fared better than bottled tea in terms of EGCG content.

→ WHERE TO BUY
Grocery stores and supermarkets.

Lipton contained the highest amounts of EGCG in the study, and Bigelow tea bags also did well. In the loose tea category, Teavana's Gyokuro Imperial contained the highest quantity of EGCG.

Licorice root extract is a medicinal herb (not to be confused with the artificial flavoring). Gaia Herbs makes an alcohol-free herbal extract that can be purchased in the herbal supplement section of stores like Whole Foods.

APPLE CIDER VINEGAR
(Toner, pH balancer and acne control)

Good for men's skin, teenagers and oily skin types. Suggested uses:

TONER Pour 1-part apple cider vinegar into a glass jar, bottle or container, add 2-parts distilled or filtered water. Shake well to combine the mixture. Does not need to be refrigerated, but do keep in cool place. Make a new batch every month or so.

Use at night, after cleansing, then continue with regular nightly routine. Apply with a cotton ball or pad, avoid contact with eyes.

MIST Follow the same directions, but combine 1-part ACV to 8-parts water. The mist may be stored in a spray bottle.

pH BALANCER If you use soap in the shower you drive skin's normal pH of 5.5 higher, since soaps are alkaline. To lower pH, lightly spray your body after a shower with the mist (8 parts dilution of ACV).

ACNE CONTROL Cleansing with a pH balanced cleanser (around 4.5 to 6) is important, and with active acne you are probably cleansing at least twice a day. However, cleansing can interfere with pH balance, and maintaining a pH that is somewhat acidic but not too acidic—ideally 4.5 to 5.5—is key to preventing future breakouts. Adding a splash of ACV to your final rinse water after cleansing helps skin return to and maintain proper pH levels very quickly. Add 1 to 5-6 tsps warm water. At night, follow cleansing and rinsing with toner.

→ WHAT TO BUY
Natural apple cider vinegar differs from distilled or refined vinegars. Natural ACV ferments in tanks, and when mature it contains a web-like substance called "mother" that becomes visible when the rich, brownish liquid is held to the light. This vinegar contains bioflavonoids that help with acne.

→ SUGGESTED BRANDS
Bragg and Eden Organic both make good apple cider vinegars, found in most supermarkets and in all health food stores.

EXFOLIATION

Exfoliation tends to be overrated as an acne treatment, and I certainly advise against using harsh scrubs that create microscopic tears in the skin, inviting microbial invasion. Two methods for exfoliating that are gentle enough to be used even nightly are 1) oil cleansing, using high omega-3 oils work such as safflower oil, or 2) AHA cleansing, using alpha hydroxy acids like lactic acid found in yogurt.

Below are some suggested ways to gently exfoliate without damaging skin. These methods are highly recommended for acne-prone adults worried about so over-drying their skin that they wind up exchanging wrinkles for their pimples.

SUNFLOWER OR OTHER OMEGA-6 OIL

People with acne often complain of skin that feels not just oily, but greasy. This indicates that the sebum produced is low in omega 6-type oils, so exfoliating

ACNE ANSWER

with grapeseed or sunflower oils is a great way to rebalance sebum production and clear congestion.

CLEAR CONGESTION Add a few drops of tea tree oil to ¾ cup safflower oil, sunflower oil or grapeseed oil and ¼ cup walnut or hempseed oil. Mix and store in glass container. It does not need to be refrigerated, but keep in a cool place. Apply ½ tsp of oil blend every evening to a clean face, massage in for 1-2 minutes, then rinse with warm to hot water.

MOISTURIZE You can follow your exfoliation routine by moisturizing with the same oil blend. Apply ¼ to ½ tsp of oil blend into cleansed, exfoliated skin and leave on overnight.

→ WHAT TO BUY
Always buy cold-pressed, unrefined oils, found in supermarkets and health food stores. Spectrum makes a very good line of organic oils.

YOGURT AND MASKS
(Safe for all skin types, especially good for rosacea-prone and mature skin)

Yogurt contains lactic acid, an alpha hydroxy acid that exfoliates gently and safely as base for most masks. You can customize the basic yogurt mask with a variety of ingredients that address your particular skin type or condition.

See examples below. Don't be afraid to innovate by using your favorite ingredients, such as honey, avocado, papaya and pineapple, to mention just a few.

BASIC EXFOLIATING YOGURT MASK Apply ½ tsp yogurt to clean face and neck, leave on 15 minutes, then rinse off. This mask is simple and gentle enough that you can use it nightly.

CUSTOM YOGURT MASKS

FOR ROSACEA Add 1 tbsp ground oatmeal and 1/8 tsp turmeric to 1 cup yogurt, mix well and store in glass container. Keep refrigerated what you don't use. Apply ½ tsp to face, leave on 10 to 15 minutes, then rinse. Use 2-3 times a week.

FOR ACNE Add 1-2 ground aspirin (salicylic acid) or 1 tsp white or black willow bark to 1 cup yogurt, mix well and store in glass container. Keep refrigerated what you don't use. Apply ½ tsp to face, leave on 10 to 15 minutes, then rinse. Use once a week.

FOR HYPERPIGMENTATION Add 1 tsp juice from freshly squeezed lemon to 1 tsp yogurt. Apply to face, leave on 10 to 15 minutes, then rinse. Use 2-3 times a week. Make this fresh each time.

AS A MITICIDE If you are plagued with *Human demodex* that you suspect are making your rosacea worse, try this. Add 1 tbsp ground mung beans or chickpea flour and 10 drops tea tree oil to 1 cup yogurt, mix well and store in glass container. Keep refrigerated what you don't use. Apply ½ tsp to face, leave on 10 to 15 minutes, then rinse. Use once or twice a week.

→ WHAT TO BUY
Items like white or black willow bark powder, mung bean or chickpea flour and oatmeal can be bought in the bulk section of natural food stores. If you can't find willow bark, salicylic acid from aspirin is fine. You want the cheap, non-buffered pure aspirin—not ibuprofen or an aspirin substitute. The generic drugstore brand that costs $2-$3 for a big bottle is the one you are after.

BENTONITE CLAY
(Good for acne, oily skin)

Bentonite clay comes from volcanic ash, and when mixed with water it rapidly swells, becoming a highly porous sponge. The sponge's negatively charged ions attract and bind positively charged heavy metal ions and toxins to it. The toxins remain bound during the removal process, so that when the clay is eventually washed off it takes with it toxins, bacteria and other impurities. A weekly mask will help clear skin and refine pores.

DIY RECIPE Mix 1 part powder with 1 part water or apple cider vinegar, apply a relatively thin layer, allow to dry for 10-15 minutes, then remove using warm water and a wash cloth.

→ SUGGESTED BRANDS
Redmond Clay or Aztec Secret Natural Clay can be found in most drug stores and natural food stores.

№ 2 SPECIALTY ITEMS and FINISHED PRODUCTS

Due to the enormous wealth of choices in the skin care arena, this list is far from comprehensive. It will, however, point you in the right direction. If your favorite products or brands didn't make the list, it's not because they aren't good, but simply because space is too limited to include all of the many excellent brands and individual products.

This guide is meant to be used more broadly as an aid to reading the ingredients labels—essential to identifying the active ingredients you need. I limit my suggestions to three products per category, from least to most expensive: $, $$, and $$$.

Also rated is the irritation potential, which is assessed by the presence of ingredients (usually preservatives) known to be common skin irritants, on a 0, 1, 2 scale.

CLEANSING

OIL-BASED CLEANSERS
(Good for acne, oily skin)

→ KEY INGREDIENTS
Omega 6-type oils such as safflower or sunflower for oily skin. Olive oil for dry skin.

DHC DEEP CLEANSING OIL

With olive oil, capryllic/capric triglycerides

http://www.dhccare.com/deep-cleansing-oil/?Kwrd=DeepCleansing
Oil&OrgID=1&gclid=CJGnrOLuwM0CFYpffgodS5QHDQ

$ / IRRITATION POTENTIAL: 2

MARIE VERONIQUE REPLENISHING OIL CLEANSER

With safflower and sunflower oils, and superoxide dismutase (SOD), a lipid-protective antioxidant

http://www.marieveronique.com/collections/cleansers/products/
replenishing -oil-cleanser

$$ / IRRITATION POTENTIAL: 0

VINTAGE TRADITION BODY BALM

Scented with tallow, olive oil and essential oils. Unscented with just tallow and olive oil. If you are a purist this is as good as it gets.

http://www.vintagetradition.com/food-renegade-special.php

$$$ (BUT LASTS A LONG TIME) / IRRITATION POTENTIAL: 0

ACNE ANSWER

CLEANSERS WITH SALICYLIC ACID

(Good for teen acne and men's skin)

→ KEY INGREDIENT
Salicylic acid

BURT'S BEES NATURAL ACNE SOLUTIONS PURIFYING GEL CLEANSER

With 1% willow bark extract

http://www.burtsbees.com/Natural-Acne-Solutions-Purifying-Gel-Cleanser/00181-00,default,pd.html

$ / IRRITATION POTENTIAL: 1

PERFECT IMAGE SALICYLIC DEEP GEL CLEANSER

With glycolic acid, salicylic acid, tea tree oil

http://perfectimage-llc.com/product/salicylic-deep-gel-cleanser-enhanced-with-green-tea-extract-and-tea-tree-oil/

$$ / IRRITATION POTENTIAL: 2

MARIE VERONIQUE TREATMENT CLEANSER

With 1% willow bark extract, 1% lactic acid, apple cider vinegar

http://www.marieveronique.com/collections/cleansers/products/treatment-cleanser

$$$ / IRRITATION POTENTIAL: 0

TREATMENT with OILS

OIL BLENDS

(Good for dry and oily skin. Benefits congested skin prone to blackheads.)

→ KEY INGREDIENTS
Safflower oil, sunflower oil, grapeseed oil, tea tree oil, argan oil,
pumpkin seed oil, black cumin, tamanu oil

JUST NATURAL MANUKA ACNE TREATMENT

With manuka oil, tea tree oil, jojoba oil, camellia seed oil, karanja oil

http://www.justnaturalskincare.com/9/acne/manuka-acne-relief.
html?gclid=CKf--saawcOCFUKUfgodG-EJEQ

$ / IRRITATION POTENTIAL: 1

LAUREL WHOLE PLANT ORGANICS BLEMISH TREATMENT

With black cumin oil, tamanu oil

https://www.laurelskin.com/product/blemish _ treatment/

$$ / IRRITATION POTENTIAL: 0

MARIE VERONIQUE TREATMENT OIL

With safflower oil, sunflower oil, pumpkin seed oil, borage oil, emu oil, black
willow bark extract, tamanu oil, argan oil

http://www.marieveronique.com/collections/acne-oily-skin/prod-
ucts/treatment-oil

$$$ / IRRITATION POTENTIAL: 0

REPAIR

AHA/BHA SERUMS
(Good for acne, breakouts; can be used all over or as spot treatments.)

→ KEY INGREDIENTS
Salicylic acid, lactic acid

PCA SKIN ACNE GEL

With 2% salicylic acid

http://www.pcaskin.com/acne-gel.html?bvstate=pg%3A2%2Fct%3Ar

$ / IRRITATION POTENTIAL: 1

RENEE ROULEAU ANTI-CYST TREATMENT

With lactic acid

https://www.reneerouleau.com/products/anti-cyst-treatment

$$ / IRRITATION POTENTIAL: 1

BIOLOGIQUE-RECHERCE LOTION P50

With lactic acid, salicylic acid

http://www.biologique-recherche.com/produit.php?pro _ id=75 &lang=us-en

$$ / IRRITATION POTENTIAL: 1

VITAMIN A SERUMS

(Good for teen acne and adult acne.)

→ KEY INGREDIENTS
Stabilized or encapsulated retinol, stabilized retinal,
stabilized retinaldehyde

IMPORTANT NOTES ABOUT RETINOIDS

WARNING Pregnant, potentially pregnant or nursing mothers should not use retinoid products.

CONSULT A DERMATOLOGIST Retinoids, used properly, are hands-down the best anti-acne and anti-aging weapon in our skin care arsenal. If your acne is severe, you may need a stronger retinoid than you can find over the counter to bring it under control. I strongly recommend consulting a dermatologist, who will guide you in choosing the correct course of action appropriate to your condition. There is no reason not to take advantage of the best that modern medicine has to offer—it's oftentimes pretty awesome.

HOW TO USE RETINOL OR RETINAL PRODUCTS You may experience dryness, redness, peeling or increased breakouts for the first few weeks of using a retinoid product. Do not be alarmed. This is called facial retinization and indicates that the retinoid is changing skin at a profound level. This is a good thing, but in order for the product to work it's important to keep to a consistent routine while these normal skin changes run their course.

The major reason people are not successful with retinoids is that they wait for symptoms they think they should not be having to subside, then they try again when the skin is "better." This just prolongs the discomfort of retinization and delays skin improvement.

SENSITIVE SKIN Yes, you can still use retinoids successfully even if your skin is sensitive. Contrary to the mythology, retinoids are anti-inflammatory and will not make your skin more sensitive. And rather than "thin" the skin they increase epidermal density by normalizing skin cell development, and dermal density by increasing deposition of collagen in the dermis. If you have sensitive skin, start slowly; use it every third night and gradually work up to every other night, but be consistent.

IF YOU REACT Irritation potentials are not rated here, as it's difficult to distinguish between allergic reactions and reactions consistent with retinoid activity. Of course, if reactions are extreme or involve swelling, serious flare-ups or rashes, then discontinue the product immediately and consult your dermatologist.

ACNE ANSWER

ENCAPSULATED RETINOL

PETER THOMAS ROTH RETINOL FUSION PM

With encapsulated retinol 1.5%

https://www.peterthomasroth.com/ProductSearch?&ProdSearchText
=retinol%20fusion&gclid=CKed58Kow80CFQ6maQodjv8G2g

$$

FUTUREDERM TIME RELEASE RETINOL

With encapsulated retinol 0.5%

https://www.futurederm.com/shop/futurederm-time-release
-retinol-0.5/

$$

MARIE VERONIQUE TREATMENT RETINOL

With encapsulated retinol 3.5%, ascorbic acid

http://www.marieveronique.com/collections/serums/products/
treatment-retinol-serum

$$$

STABILIZED RETINALDEHYDE

SIRCUITSKIN INFUSION-A

With stabilized Retinaldehyde

http://sircuitskin.com/inc/sdetail/44378/43689

$$

VITAMIN B SERUMS

(Good for sensitive and inflamed skin, adult acne, acne control through sebum regulation.)

⟶   KEY INGREDIENTS
Vitamin B3 (niacinamide or nicotinamide), pro-vitamin B5 (panthenol), vitamin B5 (pantothenic acid)

Niacinamide (vitamin B3) is a powerful anti-inflammatory, and studies show that a serum with vitamin B3 helps reduce discomfort associated with the facial retinization process. If you use a retinoid product and experience redness or peeling, a vitamin B3 cream can help alleviate the discomfort and speed up the renormalizing process.

Panthenol (pro-vitamin B5) applied to the skin results in a conversion to pantothenic acid. It is anti-inflammatory, moisturizing and deeply penetrative.

Pantothenic acid (vitamin B5) must be present to make coenzyme-A (CoA), which is needed to metabolize fats. Since proper fat breakdown is a crucial part of sebum regulation oral supplementation of B5 can help clear cases of chronic acne. Topical applications can also help maintain clear skin because B5 is penetrative and can assist, to some extent, in regulating sebum breakdown processes. Some people might experience an initial increase in acne because old congestion deep in the pores is broken up and pushed to the surface of the skin. It can cause skin dryness in some cases and is not recommended for adults concerned about wrinkles to use on it on areas where oil glands are in short supply, such as around eyes and upper lip.

SKINCEUTICALS METACELL RENEWAL B3

With 5% niacinamide

http://www.skinceuticals.com/metacell-renewal-b3-3606000400429.html

$$$ / IRRITATION POTENTIAL: 0

PAULA'S CHOICE RESIST 10% NIACINAMIDE BOOSTER

With 10% niacinamide, panthenol

http://www.paulaschoice.com/shop/collections/Resist-Anti-Aging/
treatments/ _ /Resist-Ten-Percent-Niacinamide-Booster/

$$ / IRRITATION POTENTIAL: 1

SERUMS + RETINOIDS

If you are experiencing facial retinization with a retinoid product, layer either of these serums over it to facilitate recovery by improving barrier function.

MARIE VERONIQUE TREATMENT SERUM

2% niacinamide, 1% pantothenic acid, panthenol

http://www.marieveronique.com/products/treatment-serum

$$$ / IRRITATION POTENTIAL: 0

VITAMIN C SERUMS

(Good for all skin types. If you are pregnant, about-to-be-pregnant or nursing a vitamin C, E and ferulic acid serum makes a good substitute for retinol.)

→   KEY INGREDIENTS
Stabilized ascorbic acid, vitamin E, ferulic acid

THE REAL SCOOP ABOUT VITAMIN C

EXCELLENT, BUT NOT EVERYTHING Topical ascorbic acid is a vital part of good skin care. An enzyme converts the amino acid hydroxyproline to collagen in the skin—but it requires vitamin C to do it. In short, if you are deficient in vitamin C your skin will not make collagen and you will get wrinkles.

Vitamin C is also a great antioxidant, is anti-inflammatory and inhibits melanin synthesis. However, despite its all-around greatness, don't be misled into thinking topical vitamin C alone will keep your skin in superb shape—especially as it ages. For that you need topical vitamin A derivatives as well. Retinoids are still very much the gold standard when it comes to improving and maintaining skin health, so it makes better sense to think of vitamin C as the other pole holding up your skin care tent.

STABILITY ISSUES Topical ascorbic acid is great when it works, but most of the time it doesn't because it oxidizes so rapidly in solution that there's usually not enough active vitamin C left when it reaches your skin to do much good. Its instability has led formulators to come up with solutions like vitamin C derivatives and vitamin C powders. Unfortunately, oil-soluble C derivatives like ascorbate phosphate and ascorbyl palmitate, aka ester-C, are usually too stable to have more than limited permeability and function in the skin.

Ascorbic acid powders, the ones in sprinkle or capsule form that you keep separate from the wetting agents until you are ready to use them, pose a different set of problems. As soon as you wet the powder and apply the resulting lotion to your skin the vitamin C recrystallizes, and crystallized vitamin C can't penetrate the skin. If that weren't discouraging enough, there is also a pH problem. L-ascorbic acid penetrates better at low pH, and mixing L-ascorbic acid with water results in a very low pH of around 2.2 to 2.5, which you'd think would be ideal—until you remember that the skin's acid mantle protects skin best when its pH is around 5 to 5.5. A pH too high can result in dry and irritated skin, but a too low pH can create redness, inflammation and quite often angry breakouts—even in people who don't normally break out.

The best solution appears to be ascorbic acid suspended in an anhydrous medium. A 2006 study published in the Journal of Cosmetic Dermatology found that ultrafine microcrystalline anhydrous vitamin C increased production of both type I and type III collagen.

ANTIOXIDANT SYNERGY Vitamin C and vitamin E work together, scavenging and recycling free radicals from one to the other in feedback loop fashion. Ferulic acid, another powerful antioxidant when acting on its own, works even better with vitamins C and E.

The most state-of-the-art vitamin C serum to be found at this stage of formulating knowledge appears to be a serum that contains stabilized ascorbic acid, vitamin E and ferulic acid.

VITAMIN C, E, FERULIC SERUMS

TIMELESS 20% VITAMIN C+E FERULIC ACID SERUM
With ascorbic acid, Vitamin E, ferulic acid

http://www.timelessha.com/20-vitamin-c-e-ferulic-acid-serum-1-oz/

$ / IRRITATION POTENTIAL: 1

MARIE VERONIQUE VITAMIS C+E+FERULIC SERUM
With 5% stabilized ascorbic acid, vitamin E, ferulic acid

http://www.marieveronique.com/products/vitamin-c-e-ferulic-serum

$$ / IRRITATION POTENTIAL: 0

SKINCEUTICALS C,E FERULIC
With 15% ascorbic acid, vitamin E, ferulic acid

http://www.skinceuticals.com/c-e-ferulic-635494263008.html?cgid=vitaminC-serum#start=1&cgid=vitaminC-serum

$$$ / IRRITATION POTENTIAL: 1

SUNSCREENS

(Necessary for all skin types.)

→ KEY INGREDIENT

Zinc oxide

BADGER UNSCENTED ORGANIC SUNSCREEN WITH ZINC OXIDE

With 18.6% zinc oxide

http://www.badgerbalm.com/p-462-organic-sunscreen-cream-spf30-
unscented.aspx

$ / IRRITATION POTENTIAL: 0, SPF 30

CLIMBON SPF 30 MINERAL SUNSCREEN

With 20% zinc oxide

http://skinourishment.com/collections/climbon/products/
spf-30-mineral-sunscreen

$ / IRRITATION POTENTIAL: 0, SPF 30

MARIE VERONIQUE EVERYDAY COVERAGE, SPF 30

With 20% zinc oxide

http://www.marieveronique.com/products/everyday-coverage-spf-30

$$$ / IRRITATION POTENTIAL: 0, SPF 30

№ 3 SAMPLE AM/PM ROUTINES using REAL PRODUCTS

Clara's Case Study is fully outlined on page 96.

CLARA'S ROUTINE: FIRST FOUR WEEKS

→ MORNING

Cleanse with Treatment Cleanser.

Mist with Treatment Mist.

If you want extra antioxidant protection, add your vitamin C, E, ferulic acid serum here.

Apply a few drops of Treatment Oil all over face.

Apply sunscreen.

It is not necessary for face to dry between steps.

→ EVENING

Cleanse with Treatment Cleanser.

Mist with Treatment Mist.

Apply Treatment Serum** or Retinol Serum*

Finish with Treatment Oil.

* We alternated Treatment Serum with Treatment Retinol Serum, using one or the other every other night until her skin adjusted to the retinol. After four weeks she graduated to using the retinol every night, reserving the Treatment Serum for spot treatments.

** Pregnant, about-to-be-pregnant and nursing women can safely use Treatment Serum every night.

→ WEEKLY

Clara was seeing us weekly for facials for the first four weeks, but in lieu of visits to an esthetician, weekly masks are a great way to speed up the clearing and healing process. You can apply the following clay mask 1-2 times a week.

DIY MASK Bentonite Clay makes a great mask. Redmond Clay or Aztec Secret Natural Clay can be found in most drug stores or natural food stores. Mix 1 part powder with 1 part water or apple cider vinegar, apply a thin layer, allow to dry for 10-15 minutes, then remove using warm water and a wash cloth.

Do this at night, then follow with your regular nightly routine. You can skip the serum step on the nights you use a mask if your face feels dry, but do finish with the Treatment Oil after your mask treatment to keep skin from getting too dry.

SUPPLEMENTS

→ FIRST TWO WEEKS
Vitamin B5, 500 mgs 2 x a day, and 1 multivitamin, multi-mineral capsule 1-2 x a day (more if directed on bottle)

→ AFTER TWO WEEKS
Increase supplementation of B5 to 1000 mgs 3 x a day
500 mgs acetyl carnitine 1 time a day
(Multivitamin, multi-mineral intake stays the same.)

RECOVERY

After four months, when Clara's breakouts looked like they were gone for good, we knew it was time to address the residual effects such as scarring and post-inflammatory hyperpigmentation (PIH). We introduced Lightening Serum to eliminate the last effects of her acne. It is always possible to layer serums to get speedier results, so in this case we advised Clara to use Treatment Retinol Serum followed by Lightning Serum, then layer Treatment Oil last over top to moisturize.

WHAT'S NEXT?

It's pleasant for Clara to contemplate her acne as a distant memory (unless she's reminded when someone mentions the book). In any event, she's been a great sport about it, and it probably doesn't hurt that her skin has remained clear and healthy—we just saw her about a month ago.

Her maintenance program is not too much different from the initial routine we set up for her, since skin is an organ that needs constant care and feeding.

→ THE FOUR THINGS SKIN NEVER STOPS NEEDING (JUST LIKE THE REST OF YOUR BODY):

Vitamin A

Vitamin C

Essential fatty acids from oils

Sun protection

MAINTENANCE PROGRAM

Clara keeps her skin healthy and clear with this maintenance program.

→ MORNING

Don't need to wash, splashing on a bit of tepid water is enough.

Mist with Treatment Mist.

Apply vitamin C, E, ferulic acid serum.

Apply a few drops of Treatment Oil all over face.

Apply sunscreen.

→ EVENING

Cleanse with Treatment Cleanser.

Mist with Treatment Mist.

Treatment Retinol Serum every other night; alternate with Lightning Serum on nights when not using Retinol Serum.

Finish with Treatment Oil.

INDEX

ACKNOWLEDGMENTS

It seems like no book gets written without a village, and this book in particular would not exist without the help, encouragement and support of more people than I can name here, but I do want to call out a few.

To Daniela Serra, whose esthetician's brilliance made our case study a success, and to Sara Crane for her patience and trust in us over the long haul, and for letting us use her pictures.

To another brilliant esthetician, Kristina Holey, for her continued collaboration and fascination with all things obscure and skin-related.

Lasting gratitude and thanks go to my editor, Claudia Anastasio, for her ability to turn clumsy prose into something readable, and to my publisher for her unfailing willingness to guide the book through its many iterations. My heartfelt thanks go to Hallie Overman, whose design brilliance has turned cumbersome text into a readable book, and Kristy Moore-Jeffress whose creative input on the cover made all the difference.

To my daughter, Jay Nadeau, whose microbiologist's eye at many turns in the road prevented the book from plunging over the Cliff of Error.

Heartfelt thanks to all my clients who have asked me for advice and whose stories have given me the inspiration to write this book.

Last but not least, I want to extend my appreciation and gratitude to my trillions of microbes, without whose support this book, or indeed anything else, would not have been possible.

ABOUT THE AUTHOR

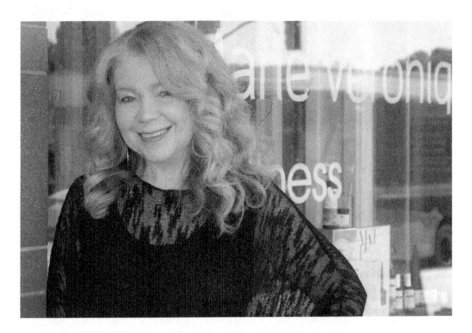

MARIE VÉRONIQUE NADEAU is the founder of Marie Veronique Advanced Skin Care (formerly Marie Veronique Organics). The company began in her kitchen lab with a groundbreaking, zinc oxide-only sunscreen for sensitive skins. Its success led to effective, nontoxic treatments for rosacea and aging skin. Now, Marie Veronique takes on acne—a challenge that has daunted the skin care world since Zorg applied mastodon grease to soften wrinkles.

Paleo skin care may make a comeback yet, but till then Marie Veronique's Darwinian approach to battling the flaming reds helps teens and adults conquer their acne when absolutely nothing else has worked.

Marie Veronique has a BS in math and chemistry, and taught high school chemistry in a former life. She is author of *The Yoga Facelift*.

CPSIA information can be obtained
at www.ICGtesting.com
Printed in the USA
FSOW03n1309230417
33338FS